PREVENTION'S
Anti-Aging
Secrets

PREVENTION'S
Anti-Aging
Secrets

HUNDREDS OF FAST & EASY WAYS TO LOOK YOUNGER & FEEL GREAT!

By the editors of

PREVENTION
Health Books™

Rodale Press, Inc.
Emmaus, Pennsylvania

—— OUR PURPOSE ——

*"We inspire and enable people to improve
their lives and the world around them."*

CONTENTS

INTRODUCTION: IT'S EARLIER THAN YOU THINK.......ix

Part I: Stopping the Age Robbers
AGE SPOTS...3
Make Them Fade Away
ARTHRITIS 6
Ways to Beat the Pain
BACK PAIN...10
Coping with a Common Ache
BURNOUT 14
Turning Down the Heat
CELLULITE 18
It's Fat—And Nothing Else
DOUBLE CHIN...21
Going Neck and Neck with Aging
FATIGUE...24
How to Restore Your Energy
FOOT PROBLEMS 27
Keeping Your Feet in Top Form
GRAY HAIR 31
Showing Your True Colors

HAIR LOSS 34
Winning over Thinning
HEARING LOSS 38
Fending Off the Sounds of Silence
HIGH BLOOD PRESSURE 42
The Silent Thief of Youth
IMPOTENCE 46
Living Well Shrinks Your Risk
MENOPAUSAL CHANGES 49
They're Bound to Happen
OSTEOPOROSIS 53
Strengthening Your Support System
OVERWEIGHT 57
Getting Yourself Down to Size
PROSTATE PROBLEMS 61
Corralling the Male Menace
STRESS 64
Control Is the Cure
TELEVISION ADDICTION 68
Pandora's Electronic Box
TYPE A PERSONALITY 71
A Is for Attitude
VARICOSE VEINS 74
You Don't Have to Live with Them
VISION CHANGES 77
Set Your Sights High
WRINKLES 81
Draw the Line on Early Lines

Part II: The Age Rejuvenators

ADVENTURE 87
Reach for Your Outer Limits
AEROBIC EXERCISE 90
Move into the Future Youthfully

AFFIRMATIONS 94
Phrases That Sing Your Praises
ALTRUISM 97
Helping Others to Help Yourself
ANTIOXIDANTS..101
The Best Defense Is a Good Offense
BREAST CARE...105
Keeping Your Breasts Firm and Healthy
CONFIDENCE AND SELF-ESTEEM 109
Be Your Own Best Friend
FIBER 112
Staying Young Inside and Out
FLUIDS 116
Life's Liquid Assets
FRIENDSHIPS...119
They're Good for Life
GOALS...122
Your Road Map to Vitality
HORMONE REPLACEMENT THERAPY....................125
A Midlife Option
HUMOR 129
It's No Joke—Laughter Is Healthy
LEARNING...133
Have It Your Way
LOW-FAT FOODS 136
Eating Lighter and Liking It
MASSAGE..140
Much-Kneaded Relief
MEDICAL CHECKUPS 143
Well Worth Your Time
OPTIMISM 148
A Proven Power for Health
RELAXATION 151
Mother Nature's Secret Life-Enhancer

RELIGION AND SPIRITUALITY 155
The Strength of an Ageless Soul
RESISTANCE TRAINING..159
Give Your Life a Lift
SEX...163
It Does a Body Good
SKIN CARE 166
Maintaining Your Youthful Look
STRETCHING...170
Get Loose, Feel Good
VITAMINS AND MINERALS....................................174
Life's Bare Necessities

INDEX..179

INTRODUCTION

It's Earlier Than You Think

Ever hear that old saying, "Getting old is tough, but it sure beats the alternative"? Sort of makes you want to throw up your hands in submission, doesn't it? Well, take heart: As scientists learn more about human potential, it's becoming clear that while growing old is inevitable—there's really no way to stop the clock—the breakdown of your body is not.

There is no such thing as the "aging process." There are no rules that say you will have trouble walking at this age or begin to lose your mental edge at that age. While you probably know people who began sliding rapidly downhill in their fifties, you also know others who are in great shape, not just "for their age" but for any age.

"Many of the changes that we blame on aging really have nothing to do with getting older," says Ben Douglas, Ph.D., professor of anatomy at the University of Mississippi Medical Center in Jackson and author of *AgeLess: Living Younger Longer*. Things such as diminished vitality and strength, mental fogginess, and premature wrinkling are not natural effects of aging that automatically occur at 40, 50, 60, or 70. All are caused by the way you live, which means that all can be controlled.

While the earlier you start to combat the effects of advancing years, the better, it really is never too late. "There is a lot of research showing that these wonderful bodies of ours are almost indefinitely renewable if we give them a chance," says Walter Bortz, M.D., clinical associate professor of medicine at Stanford University and author of *We*

Live Too Short and Die Too Long. In fact, researchers at Duke University in Durham, North Carolina, have calculated that simply by taking charge of certain key actions in your life—such as eating right and exercising regularly—you can boost your life expectancy by up to 15 years.

"The human body is designed to last 110 years," says Dr. Douglas. "Just as with other members of the animal kingdom, our bodies are designed to last roughly five times the age at which we reach our sexual maturity. And with proper care, they should."

The Biology of Aging

Scientists who study the aging process readily acknowledge that there are some aspects of aging about which we can do little. As we grow older, certain changes, called biomarkers of aging by those in the field, tend to occur.

What are these changes? Well, you can't stop your hair from graying and thinning. With time, your skin becomes looser and more wrinkled. A certain amount of degeneration is natural for your senses: vision gets fuzzier, hearing begins to fade. And yes, you lose some muscle strength. Metabolism also slows down, so you're more likely to gain weight even if you're careful not to ingest more calories. Reproductively, as hormone levels drop, women experience menopause, and men's sexual urges decrease somewhat.

Other changes are less noticeable, but they can be more significant to your overall health. Cholesterol levels start increasing steadily. Immunity weakens, so you're more susceptible to illness and take longer to bounce back. Women face the risk of osteoporosis, and men may start having prostate problems. Even brain cells start dying off by the thousands each day, starting at around age 30.

But again, on their own, none of these changes will seriously restrict your life. In fact, good lifestyle choices can reduce the chances that any of them will have significant effects on your health or vitality.

Why Do Men Die Younger?

Oddly, there is one risk factor that you have no control over that does seem to have an effect on longevity: your gender.

In the United States, and in virtually every other society, males typically die seven years earlier than females—and we're not talking only about humans. From apes to canaries to leopard frogs, "studies disclose that greater female longevity is virtually universal in zoology," says William R. Hazzard, M.D., chairman of the department of internal medicine at the Bowman Gray School of Medicine of Wake Forest University in Winston-Salem, North Carolina.

Although we can't explain why this is true for critters, researchers have some theories on the reasons that men typically die at age 72, while women generally reach the age of 79. There are several factors at work.

Smoking plays a partial role, although men now smoke less and women are smoking more. And then there's the fact that life seems to be more dangerous for men: They are twice as likely to die from an unintentional injury as women and nearly three times as likely to die from suicide or murder. And experts say that although women continue to gain more opportunities in the workplace, social expectations still encourage men to perform more hazardous jobs. This is why they are 29 times more likely than women to fall to their deaths from a ladder, 23 times more likely to be killed by machinery, and nearly 20 times more likely to be electrocuted.

The main reason that women outlive men, however, is that men get diseases earlier. Men under 50 are twice as likely to die from heart disease as women of the same age, largely because the male hormone testosterone doesn't offer the same protection against cholesterol levels as the female hormone estrogen. They are also more likely to have strokes or develop cancer or other life-threatening diseases at an earlier age.

See the Glass as Half-Full

While a large part of how long and how well we live, of course, is fate, a lot of it is up to us. We may not be able to outrun Father Time, but more and more, research seems to indicate that we can keep one step ahead of him. And one significant finding is that how we think about aging may be the most crucial factor in the *way* we age.

"It's absolutely true that you're as young as you think," says Dr. Douglas, who has studied scores of centenarians, including one man who was still vibrant and disease-free at age 110. "By having the right attitude, you'll not only live longer, you'll remain younger longer."

A case in point: In a Brown University study, researchers surveyed nearly 1,400 people over age 70 who were experiencing health problems. Those who blamed their failing health on old age had a 78 percent greater risk of dying in the near future than those who cited a specific reason not related to aging. "Once you say that a problem is due to old age, you've given up in a way," explains William Rakowski,

Ph.D., of the Center for Gerontology and Health Care Research at Brown University in Providence, Rhode Island.

"Regardless of race, religion, socioeconomic background, even their diet, in my research the people who age the best all seem to share similar characteristics," Dr. Douglas says. "They all have a good sense of humor; they don't take life too seriously. They tend to be active, having worked hard every day of their lives. And they also tend to be forward-looking people. Rather than looking back at what they've done or not done, they focus on what's ahead, whether it's the election or a baseball game or seeing their grandchildren."

It may be a matter of self-perception as well. "People who live long and healthy lives have a purpose in life; they have a reason to get out of bed each morning," says Dr. Bortz. "People who live long and productive lives don't feel old because they make themselves necessary."

To further minimize your chances of feeling old, it also helps to realize that although you may have lost some ground in some areas, you've gained much more in others. Not only will optimism help you be a little happier with the inevitable, it may also actually help you live longer.

Of course, optimists are made, not born. "The right attitude needs to be cultivated," says Dr. Douglas. "It's done by realizing that the world doesn't come to an end if your team doesn't win the pennant or if the Republicans or Democrats don't get into the White House. It's going out and running the best race you can run."

Use the Age Erasers

It's important to remember, however, that even with the right mental attitude, you can't ignore the basics of good health. You have to make smart lifestyle choices to avoid most of the conditions that make you look and feel old.

"There are obvious things that you can do to look and feel younger and live longer. Don't smoke. Exercise regularly. Eat a good diet and use alcohol in moderation," says Huber Warner, Ph.D., deputy associate director of the biology of aging program at the National Institute on Aging in Bethesda, Maryland. And, he adds, "one secret to aging well is the ability to come to grips with a decline in physical function that is real while still being able to use what you have to maintain function as well as possible."

To stay young, says Mary M. Gergin, Ph.D., associate professor of psychology at the Delaware County campus of Pennsylvania State University, "we need to liberate ourselves from outdated notions of aging. We need to be unafraid and daring and willing to take risks. And we need to be willing to break the mold of aging." Once we do, she says, we need to use the age erasers that most suit our own individual needs. Here are some of the best.

Get out and sweat. If there's anything close to a genuine youth drug, it's sweat. "There's nothing science can do for you that could be of more benefit than exercise," says William Evans, Ph.D., director of the Noll Laboratory for Human Performance Research at Pennsylvania State University in University Park and co-author of *The 10 Determinants of Aging You Can Control.*

Dr. Douglas advocates a regular exercise program that emphasizes fun over anything else to keep muscles strong and metabolism high so that calories are burned more efficiently. "Do it daily, in moderation, and pick something you enjoy so you stick with it."

In one study, men and women who participated in a yearlong walking program increased their aerobic capacities by 30 percent. In another, when elderly volunteers were put on an eight-week strength-training program, researchers found that women as old as 96 were able to increase their muscle size and strength by more than 100 percent.

Researchers have also found that weight-bearing exercises such as walking, jogging, and dancing can keep bones strong and help prevent osteoporosis. And still others concluded that exercise can prevent the age-related increases in weight, triglycerides, cholesterol, and diastolic blood pressure (the bottom number in a blood pressure reading).

How much exercise is necessary to keep your body youthful?

"For years, exercise zealots kept saying that you had to work out for 30 to 40 minutes, three times a week, in order to get any benefit," says Dr. Evans. "But there's now good evidence that fairly low-level activity is also beneficial."

Low-level means taking the stairs when you could take the escalator, he adds, or parking the car far from the entrances of malls, supermarkets, workplaces—in short, anywhere you go. It also means walking 10 minutes in the morning or at lunch and another 10 minutes around dinnertime or before bed.

"It all adds up," says Dr. Evans. And the bottom line is that it will erase many of the problems that make you old before your time.

Eat veggies for longevity. Florets of broccoli, a heap of steamed carrots, or a few ruffled leaves of kale may not seem important in the larger scheme of things. But these unassuming vegetables are actually "longevity foods"—clean-burning, high-octane fuels that can prevent many causes of premature aging.

Broccoli, brussels sprouts, carrots, and most leafy green vegetables are packed with beta-carotene, the vitamin A–producing substance that has been shown to block cancer and prevent heart attacks. Kale and other green vegetables have lots of calcium, the mineral that your body needs most to maintain its youthful bone strength. And all vegetables have almost no fat or cholesterol, which means that they can help keep age-related weight gains, high blood pressure readings, and clogged arteries at bay.

Feast on fruit. Nutrients called antioxidants—vitamins C and E and beta-carotene—have turned out to be key players in what could be described as an anti-aging diet. Available in fruits, nuts, and some vegetables, antioxidants are the body's defense against free radicals, highly reactive molecules that zing around the body and do all sorts of cellular damage. These renegade molecules are implicated in the initiation of cancer, heart disease, and even aging itself—so much so that some scientists feel that the aging process is produced largely by a lifetime of tiny cellular nicks, dents, and bumps caused by free radicals as they oxidize various cells.

As their name suggests, antioxidants provide the body with a natural defense against free radicals. That's why nutritionists frequently recommend that you eat foods rich in these nutrients.

The best sources of vitamin C are a handful or two of acerola cherries or black currants or a whole guava. Other good sources are orange juice, sweet red peppers, papayas, and cranberry juice. Beta-carotene is abundant in tropical fruits such as mangoes, guavas, and papayas.

Vitamin E is found mostly in nut oils such as hazelnut, sunflower, and almond, all of which weigh in at more than 100 calories per tablespoon. You could eat the nuts themselves, of course, but you'd have to eat so many to get sufficient vitamin E that you'd be munching all the time—just like a squirrel. As a result, many people prefer to get their vitamin E from a supplement.

The best sources of beta-carotene are carrots, spinach, broccoli, and lettuce.

Walk in the moonlight. You may call the effects of sun on your skin tanning, but dermatologists call it photoaging. That's because exposure to the ultraviolet rays in sunlight is responsible for the wrinkles, speckles, uneven pigment, and age spots that we generally attribute to aging skin. With enough exposure, the skin thickens, sags, and develops a harsh, leathery texture. And the fairer your complexion, the more extensive the damage. All of this helps make you look older than you really are.

What's more, studies have shown that long-term sun exposure increases your risk of cataracts, so too much sun can also age your eyes.

It's easy to see why experts say that you should stay out of the sun as much as possible. When you do go out, apply a sunscreen with an

SPF (sun protection factor) of 15 and always wear a hat. Wraparound sunglasses will also help shield your eyes and skin.

Avoid smoke. Smoking cigarettes is a great way to spend a lot of money to age faster, feel worse, and get sick sooner. Although smoking used to be thought of as a more significant factor in men's health problems, women smokers are now just as likely to die from lung cancer as men who smoke. And for smokers who actually inhale, there's the bonus of "smoker's face"—wrinkles at the mouth, nose, and eyes that are due to the facial contortions necessary to drag on a cigarette.

Work those neurons. The best way to keep your mind alert, your intellect sharp, and your memory keen is to keep your brain active. That's because brain cells have tiny branches that grow and spread when used—just like the roots of a plant when it's watered—or wither and die when not used. Studies indicate that when an area of the brain is used intensively, that area explodes with growth. The area of the brain devoted to understanding words, for example, is much larger in college graduates than in high school grads, probably because college-educated people spend more time working with words.

In short, keeping your mind working—by pursuing an advanced degree, reading about a wide variety of topics, learning a new language, or in any way providing your brain with mental stimulation—keeps your neural filaments jangling well into old age.

Taking Control

In the pages ahead, you will find hundreds of simple, specific steps that you can take to add active, happy years to your life. We've organized this book into two parts:

• In "Stopping the Age Robbers," we look at many of the things that can most rob you of your health, vitality, and looks—and then give lots of advice on how to foil each and every one.

• In "The Age Rejuvenators," we look at several of the best activities you can do, choices you can make, or actions you can take to add years to your life.

No complex programs. No total lifestyle makeovers. Living longer isn't a draconian New Year's resolution, offered up with good intentions, then quickly forgotten. The path to a longer, fuller, more vibrant life is making lots of right choices every day, year in and year out. With *Prevention's Anti-Aging Secrets*, you'll discover how to make the right choices each and every time, choices that can truly deliver on the promise of health and joy for as many years as you can dream.

How Long Will You Live?

The choices that you make every day about what you eat, whether you exercise, and how you deal with the stresses in your life combine with genetic factors to determine your longevity. To get an idea of your potential longevity, take the following test. Keep a running tally of your score as you answer the questions.

Family History (Choose all that apply)

1. −1 One or both parents lived beyond age 75 and did not have cancer or heart disease
2. +2 Cancer in a parent or sibling
3. Coronary heart disease before age 40 in:
   +2 One parent
   +4 Both parents
4. High blood pressure before age 50 in:
   +2 One parent
   +4 Both parents
5. Diabetes mellitus before age 60 in:
   +2 One parent
   +4 Both parents
6. A stroke before age 60 in:
   +2 One parent
   +4 Both parents

Lifestyle and Health (Choose all that apply)

7. +2 Live and/or work in a heavily air-polluted area
8. Smoking:
   −1 Never smoked or quit over 5 years ago
    0 Quit 1 to 5 years ago
   +1 Quit within past year
   +5 Have smoked more than 20 years
   +1 Smoke a pipe or cigar

9. You smoke cigarettes:
   +2 Less than one pack a day
   +3 One pack a day
   +5 Over two packs a day
10. Your alcohol use:
    −1 None or seldom
     0 Drink no more than 1½ ounces of hard liquor, 5 ounces of wine, or 12 ounces of beer a day
    +2 Three or more drinks a day
11. Your blood pressure:
    −2 Below 121/71
     0 121/71 to 140/85
    +2 141/86 to 170/100
    +4 171/101 to 190/110
    +6 Above 190/110
12. Your blood cholesterol level:
     0 190 or below
    +1 191 to 230
    +2 231 to 289
    +4 290 to 320
    +6 Over 320
13. Your HDL cholesterol level:
    −1 Over 60
     0 45 to 60
    +2 36 to 44
    +4 28 to 35
    +6 22 to 27

(continued)

How Long Will You Live?—Continued

Personality and Stress Evaluation
(Choose all that apply)

15. +2 Intensely competitive
16. +2 Angry and hostile
17. +2 Don't express anger
18. +2 Work hard without feeling satisfaction
19. +2 Hardly laugh; depressed often
20. +2 Rarely discuss problems or feelings with others
21. +2 Constantly strive to please others rather than yourself
22. −2 None of the above
23. Your weight:
    - 0 Normal or within 10 percent of normal
    - +1 Overweight by 20 to 29 percent
    - +2 Overweight by 30 to 39 percent
24. You exercise:
    - −2 Vigorously, more than 45 minutes, four to five times a week
    - −1 Vigorously, at least 30 minutes, three times a week
    - 0 Moderately, at least 30 minutes, three times a week
    - +2 Moderately, twice weekly
    - +3 Rarely or never

Your Diet (Choose all that apply)

25. −2 You eat cabbage, broccoli, cauliflower, carrots, or beans three or more times a week

26. −2 You eat high-fiber grains (whole-wheat bread, brown rice, bran cereal, etc.) almost daily

27. −2 You eat three or more servings of fruits and vegetables a day

28. +1 You go on one or two fad weight-loss diets a year

29. +2 You eat butter, cream, and cheese frequently

30. +2 You eat beef, bacon, or processed meats frequently

31. +2 You salt food before tasting

32. +2 You eat more than six eggs a week

33. +2 You eat ice cream, cake, or rich desserts almost every day

Interpreting Your Score

−16 to 0. Low risk. You should enjoy a long, healthy life free of cancer, heart disease, stroke, or diabetes. Continue your lifestyle.

1 to 34. Moderate risk. You are at some risk of developing ill health and can expect to live an average life span. Check the test to see where you can lower your risk.

35 to 60. High risk. You are at considerable risk of contracting a life-threatening illness early in life and dying sooner than you should. Use the test to see how you can lower your risk. Seek medical advice.

Over 60. Very high risk. Your health is at extreme risk, and you may die prematurely. Use this test to identify your unhealthy habits and consult your physician for further advice.

Part I

Stopping the Age Robbers

AGE SPOTS

Make Them Fade Away

Age spots, or liver spots, are those harmless brown marks that appear on your face and the backs of your hands, among other places. Their only connection to age is that it often takes decades for them to form—and they have nothing at all to do with your liver.

These unsightly blotches, also called solar lentigos, can make you feel older, though, since they commonly appear on older skin. They come in several types, and doctors say that sun damage is the cause of all of them. When unprotected skin is exposed to ultraviolet rays, whether from artificial sources such as tanning booths or from years of sun exposure, it tries to protect itself by producing an overabundance of melanocytes, the pigmented cells of which freckles are made.

Freckles and age spots are different, however, says Nicholas Lowe, M.D., clinical professor of dermatology at the University of California, Los Angeles, UCLA School of Medicine. Freckles appear when you're young, they're more numerous in the summer, and they tend to fade with age. Age spots get worse—and they don't go away.

Chemical Causes

Certain substances that come in contact with your skin may cause age spots, says Karen Burke, M.D., Ph.D., a dermatologist in private practice in New York City. Psoralens, chemicals in foods such as parsley, limes, and parsnips, can cause sun sensitivity. When you handle the foods and then go out in the sun, your skin may burn more easily where the psoralens touched it. After the little blisters from the burns heal, age spots may appear in their places.

Antibiotics such as tetracycline (Achromycin), some diuretics (water pills), and antipsychotic medicines such as chlorpromazine (Thorazine) will also cause age spots when your skin is not protected from the sun, says Dr. Burke.

Musk or bergamot oil, which are common ingredients in perfumes, lotions, aftershaves, and colognes, may give you more than a nice scent. When applied to sun-exposed areas, they can produce age spots, says Dr. Burke.

An Ounce of Prevention

You can put the little spot factories in your skin out of business right now, doctors say, but it will take vigilance to keep them from gearing up again.

Screen yourself. The best way to keep more age spots from forming is to use sunscreen. "Start using on a daily basis a sunscreen with an SPF (sun protection factor) of 15 or higher," says John E. Wolf Jr., M.D., professor and chairman of the dermatology department at Baylor College of Medicine in Houston. SPF 15, for example, means that you can stay in the sun 15 times longer before burning than you could without sunscreen.

Apply sunscreen to the backs of your hands and your face first thing in the morning, Dr. Wolf says, and keep it handy for reapplying after washing your hands. If you see any new spots, switch to a higher SPF.

Remember, though, that if you're not prepared to use sunscreen every day year-round, there's really no point in treating your age spots, Dr. Lowe says. Without daily sunscreen, "in a number of months, your skin will be back in the same shape," he cautions.

Don't be too sensitive. If your skin produces age spots readily, do you have to give up your favorite scent or skin lotion because it contains musk or bergamot oil? Not necessarily, but apply it to unexposed skin rather than to your face and neck, suggests Dr. Burke. And if you're on a sun-reactive medication, such as tetracycline, don't worry. Your daily sunscreen ritual should keep you safe from new age spots.

Wash up. Wash your hands thoroughly after handling foods that contain psoralens and apply sunscreen before going outdoors, says Dr. Burke.

Out, Out, Damn Spots

If you already have an age spot or two, the most important thing is to make sure that they're not precancerous, says Dr. Wolf. "If a brown spot pops up suddenly, or an old one suddenly changes shape, becomes raised, or bleeds, have a dermatologist look at it to be certain it's not an early melanoma," he recommends.

If your age spots are mild, there are a few home treatments you can try. Other treatments will require a visit to a dermatologist. Remember, though, that with all of these treatments, you must keep using sunscreen to prevent new age spots from forming.

Bleach them away. A hair-coloring product that's at least 30 percent hydrogen peroxide, available at drugstores, can help fade smaller age spots. The highest percentages of peroxide are found in blonde shades, such as Nice 'n Easy 97 and 98 and Ultress 24, 25, and 26. Dr. Burke suggests dabbing on the peroxide with a cotton swab. You may have to use it daily for several weeks.

Ask for an Rx. More stubborn age spots respond well to prescription creams containing hydroquinone, Dr. Burke says. Ask your dermatologist about a prescription for Melanex or Eldoquin. Another prescription spot eraser is tretinoin (Retin-A), which comes in cream or gel form. Better known for its acne- and wrinkle-removing abilities, Retin-A gradually returns skin to its normal state, and as it does so, age spots fade. It can be used in conjunction with hydroquinone at your doctor's discretion, Dr. Burke says.

Consider peeling or freezing. Your dermatologist may try trichloroacetic acid, which is often used for chemical peels and is quite effective on age spots. It would be a good choice for just a few spots that aren't too dark, says Dr. Wolf. Another alternative is freezing the spots with liquid nitrogen. With these treatments, which must be done in a doctor's office, there is some risk that the chemicals will do their job too well, leaving depigmented white spots where the age spots have been removed, he says.

Zap 'em. The laser is the state-of-the-art treatment for age spots, says Dr. Lowe. "These lasers can be set to destroy only the pigment cells. The great thing about this treatment is that in the hands of an expert, you don't run the risk of having white spots where the dark spots had been." Does the laser treatment hurt? Only about as much as the snap of a rubber band, he says. Keep in mind, though, that laser treatment is the most expensive weapon against age spots.

ARTHRITIS

Ways to Beat the Pain

More than 30 million Americans have been diagnosed with arthritis—and those are just the people who were smart enough to see their doctors about that blasted pain in their joints, tendons, and muscles. Six million more suffer quietly, paying the price for a past injury, years of carrying around an extra 20 pounds, or just bad luck.

While many of us associate this disease with people of our grandparents' age, and it's true that it's the single most common chronic condition among older Americans, arthritis can and does affect many younger people as well.

Despite its reputation for being as much a part of aging as gray hair, arthritis is an equal-opportunity deployer—of pain. "Many people aren't surprised to hear that arthritis is the leading single cause of disability in people over age 45," says Paul Caldron, D.O., clinical rheumatologist and researcher at the Arthritis Center in Phoenix. "But they are surprised to learn that it's the single leading cause of disability among people of all ages."

A Burden to Body and Mind

At best, arthritis can slow down your movements and cause some pain; at worst, it can bring agony and even severe debilitation, says Jeffrey R. Lisse, M.D., associate professor of medicine and director of the division of rheumatology at the University of Texas Medical Branch at

Galveston. Because of the pain, arthritis can affect your sleep and your sex life. It can even affect your cardiovascular health since people often become sedentary when exercise is too painful.

But arthritis ages more than just the body. "Depression is almost universal among arthritis patients," says Dr. Lisse. And a lot of people with arthritis experience what is known as learned helplessness, he says, which occurs when severe arthritis pain makes them less able to take care of themselves. They must rely on others for help with basic functions, and that is a difficult situation to deal with, mentally and emotionally.

Arthur Grayzel, M.D., vice president of medical affairs for the Arthritis Foundation, adds, "I think that society almost expects people to have arthritis when they're old, so when an elderly person limps or uses a cane, it might not surprise anyone. But when you're young and your body image is very different, the effects can be devastating. The fact is, a lot of people who have arthritis—athletes, movie stars, and others in the public eye—won't admit it because it seems to have a negative image. Having arthritis makes you seem old before your time."

Different Types, Similar Pain

Most people know that arthritis causes painful, stiff, and sometimes swollen joints. But it can also affect muscles and tendons, which may not swell but are still painful. And although there are more than 100 different forms of arthritis, the most common are osteoarthritis and rheumatoid arthritis.

Osteoarthritis is the most prevalent form, affecting 16 million Americans. It usually strikes people in their forties and fifties as a result of deterioration of the cartilage in joints from stress, overweight, or injury, which is often sports-related. "That's not to say that if you play sports, you'll get arthritis," says Dr. Caldron. "But those who have experienced repeated injury to a joint, no matter how minor, have an increased chance of getting osteoarthritis." Typical trouble spots include the fingers, feet, back, knees, and hips.

Unlike osteoarthritis, rheumatoid arthritis typically affects the entire body. It is especially painful and commonly occurs in people's twenties and thirties. "What is really sad is that many people have significant pain and loss of function, and there is nothing that they can do to prevent it since we do not yet know what causes it," says Dr. Grayzel. "It strikes women three times more often than men." Unlike osteoarthritis, rheumatoid arthritis is caused by chronic inflammation in the joints that doctors believe is related to an immunological disorder.

Winning over Pain

While you may not be able to prevent rheumatoid arthritis, you can lessen its aging effects on you. And you may be able to prevent or lessen the pain of osteoarthritis. Here's how.

Lose weight. "Being overweight is a major risk factor, especially for arthritis of the knees and hips," says Dr. Grayzel. "Even when you're in your twenties or thirties, you should try to reduce your weight close to the normal range for your height. If you're 20 percent over-weight—about 160 pounds or more for the average woman—you're a prime candidate for osteoarthritis. But any weight loss helps. If you lose just 10 pounds and keep it off for 10 years, no matter what your current weight, you can cut your risk of osteoarthritis in your knees by 50 percent."

Watch what you eat. Various studies show that food plays a cru-cial role in the severity of arthritis. Norwegian researchers discovered that patients with rheumatoid arthritis saw dramatic improvement in their conditions within one month of beginning vegetarian diets. Other scientists have found that omega-3 fatty acids, which are abundant in cold-water fish such as salmon, herring, and sardines, also ease rheuma-toid arthritis pain.

"A diet low in saturated fat and animal fat seems to be helpful," says Dr. Caldron. "Eating a lot of fresh fruits and vegetables and non-red-meat sources of fat such as fish and chicken may cause the body to produce fewer pro-inflammatory substances. That's not to say a diet will cure arthritis, but it may modify the effects of arthritis.

"Some people react to certain foods, almost like an allergy," he adds. "It may result from wheat or citrus fruits, lentils, or even alcohol. The problem is, there's no way to test for this. But if you notice a sig-nificant reaction and more pain consistently within 48 hours after eating a certain food, eliminate it from your diet."

Get physical. Regular exercise to build your muscles and increase flexibility can keep osteoarthritis at bay or lessen its effects. Exercise is also recommended for rheumatoid arthritis, although workouts should be done under a doctor's supervision and emphasize range-of-motion exercises.

"Exercise improves strength and flexibility, so less stress is placed on the joints and they can move easier and more efficiently," says John H. Klippel, M.D., clinical director of the National Institute of Arthritis and Musculoskeletal and Skin Diseases in Bethesda, Maryland. "Inactivity, on the other hand, actually encourages pain, stiffness, and other symptoms."

Weight lifting is particularly useful because it builds muscle tone, which is especially important for arthritis sufferers. Emphasize building the abdominal muscles to reduce back pain and the thigh muscles for knee pain, advises Dr. Grayzel. Aerobic activities such as running, bicycling, and swimming are also helpful for improving flexibility.

Slow down when you have to. When a joint is swollen and inflamed, continuing to use it doesn't help. "Don't exercise through the pain," says Dr. Grayzel. "Otherwise, you'll just hurt more." So even if you're on a regular exercise program, skip a day (or two) when your joints or muscles begin to hurt.

Get in gear. "A frequent cause of osteoarthritis is injury, so you should take full advantage of the various protective equipment for athletes," says Dr. Caldron. "By wearing protective gear, you'll lessen the likelihood of injuring or reinjuring joints, tendons, and muscles, thus reducing the risk of osteoarthritis." That means you should wear padding on your knees, elbows, and other possibly vulnerable areas; these pads are available at most sporting goods stores.

Turn up the heat. For immediate relief, many people find that placing warm, moist heat directly on inflamed areas helps reduce pain, says Dr. Lisse. Hot water bottles, heating pads, and hot baths help. But use heat judiciously—no more than 10 to 15 minutes at a time. And be sure to take at least a one-hour break between heat treatments. Over-the-counter analgesic balms such as Ben-Gay can also help ease pain when your joints are hot, tender, and swollen, but don't use them with heat, cautions Dr. Caldron. Together, they may cause nasty reactions such as burning and blistering.

Or chill out to prevent pain. Ice, meanwhile, is sometimes recommended to prevent pain when your joints are overworked or overused. Dr. Lisse suggests that you wrap some ice in a towel and gently apply it to your joints several times a day, 15 minutes on and 15 minutes off.

You should also practice another way to cool off by finding ways to deal with the stresses in your life. When you're tense, you hurt more. So anything that you can do to relax—whether it's listening to music, meditating, or enjoying a hobby—can help, especially when the pain is severe.

BACK PAIN

Coping with a Common Ache

You wake up. You innocently ask your body to stretch. Your back screams no. Veto that. The pain subsides. You attempt to roll over. You can't. You try to sit up. You don't. You realize you can barely move. You groan. You moan. You kick your spouse. "Honey, help pull me up. No, stop—don't pull, that hurts. Let *me* pull myself up." The agonizing truth hits: It's a bad-back day.

Been there? Felt that? That's because back pain is particularly widespread in America. In fact, it is the second most common reason (after colds and flu) for doctors' visits, according to the American Academy of Orthopaedic Surgeons. It's also the fifth leading cause of hospitalization and the third most common reason for surgery, according to Gunnar B. J. Andersson, M.D., Ph.D., professor and associate chairman of the department of orthopedic surgery at Rush-Presbyterian–St. Luke's Medical Center in Chicago.

But such frightening statistics mask an important truth: For most people, back pain can be easily avoided. The most common cause of back pain is weak muscles. As we get older, many of us get significantly less exercise. As a result, the muscles in the abdomen and back that support the spine weaken and get out of shape, says Alan Bensman, M.D., a physiatrist at Rehabilitative Health Services in Minneapolis. Weak muscles strain more easily. And most back pain is merely muscle strain—even those cases of early-morning freeze-up.

Now it's true that by the time you reach your thirties and forties, arthritis and other types of natural degeneration in the small joints of the back might begin to affect you, says Robert Waldrip, M.D., an orthopedic spine surgeon in private practice in Phoenix. This is why it's wise to see a doctor when back pain is recurrent, unusually intense, or radiating into other parts of your body. But in most cases, the muscles are the thing—keep them strong and limber, and you greatly reduce your chances of back pain.

Keeping Your Spine Sublime

Often, back pain is easily relieved without surgery or drugs, Dr. Waldrip says. In fact, 60 percent of people with acute back pain return to work within one week, and 90 percent are back on the job within six weeks. Here are some tips for preventing and treating back pain.

Do an early-morning stretch. "I tell my patients to always start their days by stretching while they're still in bed," Dr. Bensman says. "You've been lying prone for eight hours, and if you jump right up, you may be looking at a sore back." Before you get up, slowly stretch your arms over your head, then gently pull your knees up to your chest one at a time. Roll to the side of the bed and use your arm to help yourself sit up. Once you're sitting, put your hands on your buttocks and slowly lean back to extend your spine.

Walk away from it. Walking strengthens the postural muscles of the buttocks, legs, back, and abdomen. Try a brisk stroll or other aerobic exercise, such as swimming, bicycling, or running, for 20 minutes a day, three times a week, says Dan Futch, D.C., chief of the chiropractic staff at Group Health Cooperative HMO in Madison, Wisconsin.

Take a break. Sitting puts more strain on your back than standing. If you must sit for long periods—at work or when traveling—change position often. If possible, stand up and walk around every hour or so, says Augustus A. White III, M.D., professor of orthopedic surgery at Harvard Medical School and author of *Your Aching Back*.

Let your legs do the work. When you lift something—regardless of its weight—bend your knees, keep your back straight, and lift with your legs. "The legs are much stronger than the back and can lift a lot more weight without strain," Dr. Futch says.

Turn your back on heavy lifting. If you can't find someone to help you move a heavy object, try this maneuver as a last resort: If the object is at table height, turn your back to it, then drag or lift it. You can also use this technique for raising windows. It forces you to use your legs for leverage and reduces the pressure on your spine.

Straighten up. Maintaining good posture is one of the best ways to prevent back pain, Dr. Futch says. To improve your stance, stand against a wall or sit in a straight chair. Make sure that your shoulders and buttocks touch the wall or chair, then slip your arm into the space behind your lower back. If there's a point where your hand isn't touching both your back and the wall or chair, tilt your hips to eliminate the extra space. Hold that position for a count of 20 while checking your posture in a mirror. Also try to sense what it feels like so that you can maintain it for the rest of the day. Do the exercise once a day for three weeks to ensure that good posture becomes a habit.

Check your mattress. Your mattress should provide proper support, be level, and not sag. So if you feel as if you're sleeping in the middle of a pita bread, it's probably time to get a new mattress, says Joseph Sasso, D.C., president of the Federation of Straight Chiropractors and Organizations.

Don't be a heel. High heels change a woman's gait, which puts additional stress on the lower back and adversely affects posture, Dr. Bensman says. "High heels should be worn only for special occasions. For daily wear, heels should never exceed 1½ inches," he says. If you occasionally wear higher heels, wear them for no more than two hours at a time and always have a pair of tennis shoes or flats handy to slip into.

Roll it up. A lumbar roll, a round foam-rubber pad that's available at most medical supply stores, can help maintain the natural curve in the lower part of your spine and prevent pain in the small of your back, says Hamilton Hall, M.D., director of the Canadian Back Institute in Toronto. Whenever you sit, place the roll between your lower back and the chair.

Heed the no-smoking signs. Smoking decreases blood flow to the back and can weaken disks, Dr. Bensman says. Obviously, for smokers, the best advice is to quit.

Build your bones. Women in their thirties and forties who exercise regularly and have calcium-rich diets are less likely to suffer from back pain caused by osteoporosis later in life, Dr. Bensman says. An eight-ounce glass of skim milk, one cup of nonfat yogurt, and a half-cup of cooked broccoli a day will supply about 800 milligrams of calcium. Other good sources include salmon, sardines (with bones), cheese, buttermilk, and kale. If, like many women, you eat few calcium-rich foods, talk to your doctor about supplements.

Do the big chill. If you've injured your back, apply ice as soon as possible to reduce pain and swelling, Dr. Bensman says. Wrap an ice pack in a pillowcase or towel to protect your skin from the cold and put it on the sore spot for 10 minutes each hour until the ache subsides.

Then warm it up. Once the ice relieves any swelling—usually within 48 hours—you can begin using heat to increase blood flow to the injured area and help improve your mobility, Dr. Bensman says. Apply a warm (skin-temperature) washcloth to your back for 5 to 10 minutes every hour or take a warm 15-minute shower or dip in a whirlpool.

Put your feet up. When minor back pain strikes, lie on the floor and raise your lower legs on a chair so that your thighs are at a 90-degree angle to your hips and your calves are at a 90-degree angle to your thighs. This position relaxes key back muscles and is one of the least stressful for your spine, Dr. White says.

Keep moving. Although lengthy bed rest was once recommended for back pain, doctors now believe that the more active you are, the sooner you'll recover. In fact, two weeks of bed rest weakens muscles and the spine, which can actually slow recovery and increase chances of a relapse, Dr. Hall says. So don't stay in bed for more than two days, and while you're laid up, be sure to get up at least once an hour to walk or stretch.

Check out chiropractic. An analysis of 25 studies of spinal manipulation—the cornerstone of chiropractic treatment—found that it provides at least some short-term relief for uncomplicated, acute back pain. In a typical case, a chiropractor may do a series of thrusts with the heels of his hands along the troubled area of your spine. Ask your doctor for a referral.

Get a second opinion. More than 400,000 surgeries are done each year to relieve back pain, according to the American Academy of Orthopaedic Surgeons. Yet a Blue Cross and Blue Shield study found that almost 13 percent of spine operations are performed for inappropriate reasons. Get at least one other opinion if your doctor has suggested surgery, Dr. White says.

BURNOUT

Turning Down the Heat

You're cranky and depressed. Everything irritates you. You spend your time fighting a losing battle with fatigue, and your body has become a playground for all manner of aches and pains.

What's going on? Did you go to bed one night and age 30 years in your sleep? Obviously not. It's more likely that you have burnout, a kind of stress/boredom/frustration cocktail that can leave you feeling tired, irritable, achy, and old.

"Burnout can certainly make you feel old before your time," says C. David Jenkins, Ph.D., professor of preventive medicine and community health at the University of Texas Medical Branch at Galveston. "But luckily, burnout does not necessarily age people or take years off their lives in a permanent fashion. It can be reversed."

If you want to stop feeling decades beyond your biological age, you first need to know what has happened, and why.

No Variety, No Spark

While burnout was once thought to be almost exclusively a male issue, women's increasing responsibilities have made it a unisex problem. For either gender, however, and contrary to common belief, doing too many things is not the culprit. Instead, it's a lack of diversity that may do you in.

According to Faye Crosby, Ph.D., professor of psychology at Smith College in Northampton, Massachusetts, and author of *Juggling*, variety

14

is a basic human need and a good way of vaccinating yourself against burnout. But doing different activities is not enough: They have to answer different needs. "At work, for instance, our activities tend to be very agenda-oriented," notes Dr. Crosby. The problems start when there's too much agenda and not enough emotional outlet. And it's a setup that's all too familiar—for both men and women.

"For the most part, if you ask a man to tell you about himself, he'll tell you what he does for a living rather than about his family or hobbies," notes Herbert J. Freudenberger, Ph.D., author of *Burnout: The High Cost of High Achievement* and the originator of the term *burnout*. And while any woman in any role can burn out, it seems that those who tackle the responsibilities of both career and home are most susceptible.

Perfectionism Can Hurt

Closely related to lack of variety is the quest for perfection. "Many times, the men who suffer from burnout are the perfectionists who cannot delegate," says Dr. Freudenberger. "They give themselves absolutely no latitude when it comes to making mistakes. But to be a perfectionist is to make unrealistic demands on yourself and to set impossible goals. You might be able to do it for a while, but in the long run, burnout is almost a certainty." And, he says, for women, the chief offender is the ideal of "the perfect wife, mother, and professional. It's a concept that was widely disseminated in the 1970s and 1980s, and although I'm seeing less and less of it today, there are still many women who buy into this false belief."

The pursuit of perfection is not without its costs. One of the highest burnout ratios to be found is among air traffic controllers, who work under conditions that make anything less than perfect performance a matter of potential catastrophe. So great is the pressure not to make mistakes that many leave their jobs by the time they reach their midforties, says Dr. Jenkins, who participated in a definitive study of air traffic controllers and burnout.

But not everyone who suffers from burnout is operating in an environment that demands such perfection. Some people do it to themselves simply by setting impossibly high goals and viewing all harmless mistakes as catastrophes.

Take a Look at Yourself

How do you know if you're burned out? One way is to pay attention to your friends if they say that you've changed recently. Another is to listen to your body. "One of the first signs we noticed in the air traffic controllers who were burning out was a sense of fatigue," says Dr. Jenkins. "And I'm talking about a pervasive mental and physical fatigue that a good night's sleep will not get rid of."

Chest pain, gastrointestinal problems, headache, sleep disturbances, back pain, and a higher incidence of minor illnesses such as colds are some of the body's other responses to burnout. So are skin disorders, adds Dr. Freudenberger.

On the mental front, a lack of resilience can be a harbinger of burnout. "Our air traffic controllers called it bounce-back," says Dr. Jenkins. "They couldn't bounce back from a taxing period of heavy controlling and face the next period of activity with any sense of ease, comfort, and casualness. They were drained."

Irritability and depression are also possible. "More interesting is the development of a super-person personality," notes Dr. Freudenberger. "The person feels that he can handle everything, needs no help, and may actually become arrogant about it."

The Solution

Whether you already feel like a cranky Methuselah on a bad day or you just want to make sure you never get to that point, the following tips will help you ban burnout from your life.

Diversify. "Just as a bank must diversify its holdings so that it doesn't have to depend on one source for its profits, people have to diversify their emotional portfolios," says Dr. Crosby. "This means looking at your activities and making sure that you participate in some that are goal-oriented and some where the aim is to feel good and have fun."

Be realistic. Stop trying to be Mr. or Ms. Perfect. The trick is to give yourself a little leeway when you can. "Take stock of your situation and see what mistakes you can and can't make," says Dr. Crosby. "In other words, don't sweat the small stuff." And that goes for all activities, work-related and otherwise.

Know your needs. "If you know that you need positive feedback to replenish yourself, don't just ignore that fact," counsels Dr. Freudenberger. "Actively solicit feedback from family and friends and in the workplace." Or find people with whom you can share your feelings, achievements, and gripes. Also, don't be afraid to ask for help when you're facing tasks that could be overwhelming to handle alone.

Volunteer. "Volunteering is a very important anti-burnout device," says Dr. Crosby. "Whether you're at work or at home, you have to drop what you're doing, mentally change gears, and go interact with a whole new set of people in a whole new environment."

"It doesn't matter if you work in a soup kitchen twice a week, collect clothes, or deliver meals. You receive gratification that you are doing something for someone else," adds Dr. Freudenberger. "You may also receive some very important perspective on your life by seeing those less fortunate than you."

Take 15. "You also have to set aside some relaxation time during the course of the day," says Dr. Freudenberger. "And I mean every day, both at work and at home. When people tell me that they can't do that, I make them actually take apart their days piece by piece, and they suddenly find all sorts of little opportunities for 15-minute breaks. And that's all it really takes."

Make a getaway. Dr. Crosby prescribes a five-day vacation alone at least once a year. It's important to get away not only from your job but also from home. That means leaving your spouse, your kids, the dog, the goldfish—everything—behind. They'll get along just fine without you for five days.

Stop trying to be a superhero. "The trick is to allow yourself the occasional mistake—to recognize pressure release points where mistakes will not mean the end of the world," Dr. Crosby says. In other words, mismatched silver at the dinner party that you're throwing isn't going to signal the end of civilization. And handing in that report a day late probably won't push the company into bankruptcy.

CELLULITE

It's Fat—And Nothing Else

Life is not always fair in love and cellulite.

"Ninety-nine percent of women develop at least some dimply fat after age 30," explains Donald Robertson, M.D., medical director of the Bariatric Nutrition Center in Scottsdale, Arizona.

It wouldn't be so bad if men were sagging and bagging right along with women. But they're not. Men tend to gain weight around their midriffs rather than in their hips, thighs, and butts. Men's skin is also thicker and more elastic, so it holds the fat beneath it more firmly. Finally, fibers that anchor skin to muscle are structured differently in men than in women: Fibers that support women's skin run in only one direction, while men have tight, crisscrossed fibers that form a net to keep their fat firmly in place.

For women, much of cellulite is simply due to aging. Sometime in a woman's thirties, a natural drop in estrogen levels, along with sun damage accumulated over the years, causes the skin to lose its elasticity, says Ted Lockwood, M.D., assistant clinical professor of plastic surgery at the University of Missouri at Kansas City School of Medicine. The skin sags a little here, bags a little there. At the same time, the supporting network of fibers that anchor the skin to the underlying muscles starts to stretch. That, combined with the extra pounds that most of us put on as we approach midlife leads to cellulite, which is just a fancy word for what is really just dimply fat and skin that has lost its elasticity.

What to Do about It

As with other forms of fat, you can dump cellulite. Here's how.

Work it off. Women who try to get rid of cellulite by doing exercises for only the thighs and buttocks fail miserably. "Spot reducing doesn't work," says Susan Olson, Ph.D., director of psychological services at the Southwest Bariatric Nutrition Center in Tempe, Arizona. The best way to reduce cellulite—as with fat anywhere else on your body—is with aerobic activity that burns calories throughout the entire body. The best activity is one that gets your heart rate up and keeps it there for 20 continuous minutes at least three times a week. Running, walking, bicycling, skating, dancing, and swimming, all of which stoke up the metabolism for efficient fat burning, are perfect.

Just remember, however, if you've led a sedentary life, check with your doctor before embarking on any exercise program.

Pump some iron. A good aerobic workout will help tone muscles. But building them up through weight training may also help hide dimpled skin. "Bulking your muscles can make a slight improvement," says Dr. Lockwood. "Just don't expect miracles." Check with a trainer at your gym for a program that will help you.

Ditch the fat in your diet. Besides exercise, eating a low-fat diet is the best way to keep cellulite to a minimum. "A lot of cellulite comes from eating high-fat foods," says Maria Simonson, Sc.D., Ph.D., professor emeritus and director of the Health, Weight, and Stress Clinic at the Johns Hopkins Medical Institutions in Baltimore. "So the less fat you have in your diet, the less problem you'll have."

Try limiting your total fat intake to around 25 percent of calories, adds Dr. Simonson. You can track fat intake by reading product labels and staying away from high-fat fare such as cakes, cheeses, fried foods, and processed luncheon meats.

Knuckle under. "A deep massage using the knuckles may help break up the dimples," says Dr. Robertson. When combined with weight loss and smart eating, a twice-weekly massage helps whittle down the most resistant fat pockets.

Cream it. Rubbing any skin cream that contains alpha hydroxy acids—essentially, acids made from fruits or milk—into your skin will give your body a smoother look. But remember: No cream or lotion will get rid of cellulite.

Camouflage it. Use a tanning cream to camouflage cellulite. The darker color will even out your skin tone and make the shadows cast by the lumps of fat beneath the skin less apparent.

Smear on the sunscreen. You can't undo the years of sun exposure that paved the way for cellulite by zapping your skin's elasticity. "But by limiting your sun exposure or using a good sunscreen when you're outdoors, you can keep your skin from degenerating further," says Dr. Lockwood. The sun's skin-damaging rays are most harmful between 10:00 A.M. and 2:00 P.M., so it's essential to keep your thighs and other vulnerable areas covered during those hours. And whenever you're in the sun, be sure to use a sunscreen with a sun protection factor (SPF) of at least 15.

Consider a nip and tuck. If all else fails and you feel that cottage-cheese thighs are ruining your life, there is one surgical procedure that may be able to reduce your cellulite, says Dr. Lockwood. By performing nip-and-tuck surgery—which costs several thousand dollars and is generally not covered by health insurance—a plastic surgeon can stretch the skin of problem areas to hide the fatty deposits underneath. As with any surgery, consider your practitioner's experience and reputation. You may want to get a second opinion before proceeding.

DOUBLE CHIN

Going Neck and Neck with Aging

Mother Nature didn't do us any favors when she invented gravity. Since the day we slipped off our prom dresses and tuxedos, it's been tugging, tugging, tugging on us, pulling body parts to places that we would never have thought possible in our teens.

And of all our body parts, none is more gravity-sensitive than the neck. Add a few innocent pounds, a few harmless years, and—aarrgh!—here comes a double chin.

"I must say, a double chin makes some people feel like they're aging in a hurry," says Robert Kotler, M.D., a facial cosmetic surgeon and clinical instructor in surgery at the University of California, Los Angeles. "Every time they look in the mirror, they see it. And it's telling them that maybe they're not as young as they used to be."

Jaw Droppers

Three factors contribute to double chins: body fat, anatomy, and time. If we gain a few extra pounds, there's a good chance that some of that weight will settle under our chins, says Dr. Kotler.

But overweight people aren't the only ones in danger. Even thin people get double chins, usually because of the shape of their jaws and throats. "The less sharp the angle between the jawline and neckline, the greater the risk of a fleshy neck," says Dr. Kotler. But the lower your Adam's apple is in your neck, the more likely you are to get a sag in your chin.

Age also increases the odds. Women's skin starts to lose its elasticity after 35 to 40 years. For men, it's after 40 to 50 years. Even if you're fit and firm, you may still show a slight double chin simply because your skin is looser, Dr. Kotler says.

From a health perspective, none of this really matters. There's nothing dangerous about a double chin unless you're seriously overweight, Dr. Kotler says.

Keeping Your Chin Up

Harmless or not, most people still find double chins unattractive. To help get rid of those extra folds, or at least to hide them a little, experts offer these tips.

Drop 10. Or maybe 15 or 20—pounds, that is. "The single best way to get rid of a double chin is to lose weight," Dr. Kotler says. "Lots of people come to my office wanting cosmetic surgery. But if they just take off some excess weight, the problem usually diminishes to the point where they don't need any more help."

The standard rules apply. Get regular aerobic exercise. Eat less fat. Avoid crash diets, which usually do more harm than good. And don't rely on miracle spot-reducing exercises for your neck. They won't remove the fat, and in some cases, they have caused dislocated jaws and severely strained neck muscles.

Get cropped. For women, long hair draws attention to the neck, which is precisely what they should avoid. Pageboy cuts that curl under the chin are the worst. "The rule is to keep it short, at or above the jawline," says Kathleen Walas, fashion and beauty director for New York City–based Avon Products and author of *Real Beauty...Real Women.*

For men, long hair—on the head or face—is also no good. "Hair at or below your jawline is only going to make things worse," says Walas. That means no shoulder-length hairstyles. Neatly trimmed mustaches and beards are okay.

Make up the difference. Women can play down a double chin by playing up another feature. Walas suggests using blush high on your cheekbones. Or try a brighter, tasteful shade of eye shadow. If you use foundation, apply it one shade darker under your chin and blend it carefully with the foundation on your face. "That will make the rest of your face bright and attractive and your double chin much less noticeable," Walas says.

Let your neck breathe. Open, broad necklines are more flattering for women with double chins, Walas says. Turtlenecks are a definite no-no. As for jewelry, avoid chokers and try longer necklaces. Dangling earrings—anything below the jawline—can bring attention to your neck, according to Walas.

Nothing exposes a double chin on a man more than a dress shirt that is too tight around the neck. "You start to look like a stuffed sausage," says G. Bruce Boyer, a New York City fashion consultant and author of *Eminently Suitable*. Swallow your pride and buy a bigger size. And avoid spread, round, and pin collars, as they only accentuate your neck. With casual shirts, try open collars and stay away from turtlenecks. The darker the color around the neckline, the better.

Know your knots. Silk ties are better than bulky knit or wool ones, Boyer says. And never use the oversize Windsor knot to tie them. A four-in-hand or half-Windsor knot produces a neater, smaller look that doesn't draw people's eyes to your neck.

Know the skinny on surgery. Cosmetic surgery is a last resort, Dr. Kotler says. But if you have tried everything else and can't lose that extra chin—and have about $4,500 handy—you can have your neck "sculpted." The surgeon will make a small horizontal cut under your chin, then suck out the fat that has collected beneath the skin. Finally, he will make a vertical incision between the layers of the neck and jaw muscle and sew the edges together, tightening the muscle layer like a corset.

It's a relatively painless procedure that requires two adhesive bandages to hide, Dr. Kotler says. Bruising is minimal, and within about 10 days, you won't see anything except your old single chin. "It's a common procedure," he says. "The technique has become very refined, and the results are quite good." The operation can be done under either general anesthesia or local anesthesia with sedation.

For an extra $500 or so, the surgeon can add a chin implant. It's a piece of solid silicone that is slipped between your jawbone and the sheath of tissue that covers the bone. The implant gives you a more prominent jaw and further accentuates the angle between your jawline and neck, Dr. Kotler says. There is no addition to overall recovery time. Surgeons use implants in about one-fourth of all double-chin procedures, he says.

FATIGUE

How to Restore Your Energy

Ever wonder why your get-up-and-go has gotten up and gone? Blame fatigue.

We feel weak. Our bodies ache. Our spirits sag. And before we know it, we've been transformed from active, vibrant lovers of life into washed-up, worn-out zombies who feel 100 years old.

"When you don't have the strength or energy to move, even simple tasks become difficult," says Lt. Col. Kurt Kroenke, M.D., associate professor of medicine at the Uniformed Services University of the Health Sciences in Bethesda, Maryland, and an expert on fatigue. "For some, this persistent weariness can be so debilitating that they can't even get out of bed."

Fatigue can take a toll on your mind as well, experts agree. Thinking becomes difficult and confused. Decisions come slowly. Even your outlook on life turns gloomy. Your work suffers, and you spend less time with family and friends.

Recharge Your Batteries

Fatigue is a symptom of everything from the common cold to cancer. The list also includes hepatitis, diabetes, heart disease, tuberculosis, thyroid problems, Hodgkin's disease, multiple sclerosis, anemia, AIDS, anxiety, and depression.

But fatigue is rarely anything to worry about unless it's accompanied by pain, swelling, or fever or lasts longer than a week. These are signals to see your doctor. Otherwise, here are some re-energizing tips.

Pace yourself. "Fatigue is the price we pay for pushing ourselves beyond the point where our minds and bodies say no," says Dr. Kroenke. Avoid pushing yourself past your natural limits. Don't work or exercise as hard, as fast, or as long. Take frequent breaks. And make sure you get a good night's sleep every night so you wake up refreshed.

Avoid needless worry. Agonizing over situations beyond your control only eats up personal energy, says Thomas Miller, Ph.D., professor of psychiatry at the University of Kentucky College of Medicine in Lexington. Learn to let go of things that you cannot change and focus your energies on those that you can.

Clear the clutter. Does a list of tasks leave you feeling zapped before you even begin? Attack tasks bit by bit, says exercise physiologist Ralph LaForge, instructor of health promotion and exercise science at the University of California, San Diego. Start your day with a list of four or five tasks that you can definitely accomplish and work only on them. The next day, try four or five more. What seemed like a mountain of work that you couldn't climb becomes a series of small hills.

Make time for play. A steady routine of nothing but work puts more stress on the mind and the body than they can handle, says Dr. Miller. Including enjoyable activities and social events each day gives you a needed break from work and energy-draining stresses.

Hit the road. A brisk 10-minute walk causes a shift in mood that quickly raises energy levels and keeps them high for up to two hours, according to a study by Robert Thayer, Ph.D., professor of psychology at California State University, Long Beach.

Counteract the energy drop you experience after eating a big meal by taking a stroll, adds Peter Miller, Ph.D., executive director of the Hilton Head Health Institute, a clinic in South Carolina. Digesting large meals increases blood and oxygen flow to the stomach and intestines, and this draws energy away from muscles and the brain. But a walk will keep blood and oxygen circulating evenly throughout the body.

Eat the right foods. A junk-food diet high in sugar, fat, and processed foods gives your body few or none of the basic vitamins, minerals, and nutrients that it needs to perform at normal levels.

Ideally, every day you should be getting 60 percent (or more) of your calories from carbohydrate-rich foods such as pasta, bread, potatoes, and beans; 25 percent (or less) of your calories from the fat found in foods such as canola oil, olive oil, and peanut butter; and 15 percent of your calories from protein-rich foods such as chicken and fish, says Dr. Peter Miller. Of the three energy-supplying nutrients, carbohydrates pack the best fatigue-fighting punch because they provide an efficient, long-lasting energy source, he says.

Eat more frequently. Skipping meals can leave your fuel reserves dangerously low, and digesting big meals can be an enormous energy drain. Unfortunately, the traditional three meals per day may contribute to the problem.

"Your body needs fuel in moderate doses throughout the day to keep performing at optimal levels," says Dr. Peter Miller. He recommends eating four or five small meals each day.

Snack wisely. When your stomach's growling and your energy's waning, the best pick-me-ups are of the natural variety, says Dr. Peter Miller. Fruits, raw vegetables, nuts, and unbuttered popcorn—all of which are low in energy-draining fat—are excellent energizers.

Avoid a sugar fix. Sugar-loaded foods such as candy and soda may zip up your energy level for a while, but they also cause blood sugar levels to increase and then drop sharply. Unfortunately, the result is that your energy level will dip even lower than it was before, says Dr. Peter Miller.

Drink coffee. Researchers at the Massachusetts Institute of Technology have discovered that the caffeine in a single cup of coffee can boost your energy level for up to six hours. But don't overdo it.

Stay wet. Feeling run-down is often the first sign of dehydration, says Dr. Peter Miller. Drinking at least six glasses of water a day—more if you're active or dieting—will prevent this type of fatigue.

Avoid booze and pills. Regular use of alcohol, sleeping pills, and tranquilizers will make anybody act like a zombie, says Dr. Kroenke. And believe it or not, stimulants and pep pills can take you from way, way up to way, way down after their immediate effects have worn off.

Check your medicine cabinet. Antihistamines and alcohol, both of which are found in a wide variety of over-the-counter and prescription cold medications, can make you feel groggy, says Dr. Kroenke. Ask your doctor or pharmacist to recommend a nonfatiguing alternative.

Explore alternative approaches. Many people fight fatigue by going beyond the traditional limits of Western science, says LaForge. Meditation, yoga, and massage are just a few of the nontraditional options that practitioners say will energize, refresh, and revive both body and mind. Check your local telephone directory for organizations that teach these techniques.

Ask your doctor about supplements. In addition to a balanced diet, a multivitamin/mineral supplement should ensure that you're getting all the vitamins and minerals that you need, says Dr. Kroenke. Talk to your doctor about which one is right for you.

FOOT PROBLEMS

Keeping Your Feet in Top Form

Each step we take—from chasing a Frisbee to climbing the ladder of success at work in high heels or wing tips—moves us one step closer to possible foot problems.

When our poor dogs howl in pain, it can hurt all over. "Bad feet can throw your posture out of whack, setting you up for possible knee pain, hip pain, back pain, and neck pain," says Marc A. Brenner, D.P.M., a podiatrist in private practice in Glendale, New York.

Even our psyches get their share of misery. "Debilitating foot problems make you feel older by robbing you of the vigor or energy you once had," says Glenn Gastwirth, D.P.M., deputy executive director of the American Podiatric Medical Association.

But it doesn't have to be that way. With a little know-how, you can dance around foot problems and breathe new life into tired tootsies.

Foot and Heel Pain

There are several causes of those "unexplained" pains in your foot or heel. They include fallen arches, Achilles tendon stiffness, plantar fasciitis (inflammation in the bottom of the foot), and heel spurs (tiny bone growths that may result from the constant pulling of ligaments through jumping, walking, or running). No matter what the cause, though, here are some solutions.

Seek support. "Wearing high-quality, supportive, cushioning insoles or heel cups in your shoes can certainly ease some of your discomfort," says Philip Sanfilippo, D.P.M., a podiatrist in private practice in San Francisco. The inserts can help prevent excess movement and ease pain.

Stretch out your calf. Many people find relief by stretching the heel cord, or Achilles tendon, on the back of the foot, says Gilbert Wright, M.D., an orthopedic surgeon in private practice in Sacramento, California. Stand about three feet from a wall and place your hands on the wall. Lean toward the wall, bringing one leg forward and bending your arms at the elbows. Your back leg should remain straight, with the heel on the floor, so you feel a gentle stretch.

Roll away pain. For heel spurs and plantar fasciitis, try massaging the bottom of your foot. "Roll your foot from heel to toe over a rolling pin, a golf ball, or even a soup can," advises Richard Braver, D.P.M., sports podiatric physician for several New Jersey university teams. "This eases pain by stretching out the ligaments."

Heat your feet in the morning. "If you feel stiffness in your foot when you wake up, heat it to stimulate blood flow," says Dr. Braver. He recommends placing a warm compress or hot water bottle on the bottom of your foot for about 20 minutes.

Ice them at night. Place an ice pack on your foot for 20 minutes at night, remove it for 20 minutes, and then reapply it for 20 minutes, suggests Suzanne M. Tanner, M.D., assistant professor in the department of orthopedics at the University of Colorado Sports Medicine Center in Denver. Be sure to wrap the ice in a towel to prevent ice burns or frostbite.

Corns and Calluses

Corns are lumps of built-up dead skin that form on the bony areas of your feet, such as the toes. They're caused by friction, usually the result of wearing shoes that are too tight. Calluses are essentially corns on nonbony places. Both can make you feel as though you're walking on pebbles. For mild to moderate problems, try these remedies.

Make sure the shoe fits. "If you have well-fitting shoes, you usually won't have corns and calluses," says Jan P. Silfverskiold, M.D., an orthopedic surgeon in private practice in Wheat Ridge, Colorado, who specializes in foot problems.

For proper fit, have both your feet measured for length and width each time you shop for shoes, he advises. Be aware that the shape of your foot influences the best style of shoe to purchase. "Women who must wear heels," Dr. Gastwirth adds, "should buy shoes with wide, stable heels that don't exceed two inches. Look for comfort-type pumps that provide greater cushioning for shock absorption."

Apply a moisturizer. Since corns and calluses result from excessive friction, it's best to keep your skin soft and well-moisturized. Apply a moisturizer to your feet immediately after a bath or shower, recommends Suzanne M. Levine, D.P.M., adjunct clinical instructor at New York College of Podiatric Medicine in New York City and author of *My Feet Are Killing Me*. For skin that's already hardened with corns and calluses, try scraping it with an emery board or a pumice stone anywhere from daily to twice a week, adds Dr. Silfverskiold.

Be careful with the remover. Over-the-counter corn and callus removers contain salicylic acid, which will erode the lumpy lesions on your feet. But be careful: These medications should be applied only to the affected area, since they can burn healthy skin, Dr. Levine says. But don't use products containing salicylic acid if you have diabetes or poor circulation, she cautions.

Blisters and Bunions

Blisters are painful, fluid-filled separations in the skin that usually occur because of excessive friction. Bunions are bumps of bone and thickened skin on the side of your foot just below the base of your big toe. They can be accompanied by splaying of the foot and drifting of the big toe toward the little toe. Tight shoes, arthritis, and heredity can all lead to bunions. Here's how to fix either problem.

Pamper or pop 'em. If you have blisters between your toes, inserting moleskin or even little balls of cotton can bring relief and prevent them from recurring. Using cushioned insoles in your shoes may help blisters on other parts of your foot. When a blister becomes too large to pad, however, pop it by pushing the fluid to one end of the bubble and pricking that area with a needle that's been sterilized with a flame or rubbing alcohol. Repeat the procedure 12 hours later, then again 12 hours after that to ensure that you've removed all the liquid, advises Rodney Basler, M.D., a dermatologist and assistant professor of internal medicine at the University of Nebraska at Omaha. Don't pull off the skin, but if it has been rubbed off, wash the sore with hydrogen peroxide or soap and water and apply an antibiotic ointment.

Try a splint. Bunion pain can be relieved with a toe-straightening splint that's available at most drugstores without a prescription. The most common version is a rubber plug that "pulls" the big toe away from the second toe, easing pain. While moleskin pads are often used by bunion sufferers, they're not as effective as these splints.

Athlete's Foot

You can pick up this fungus, which leaves the skin on your feet scaly, itchy, cracked, and reddened, just about anywhere, but especially in warm, moist areas such as locker rooms (hence the name). Over-the-counter medications are the preferred treatment, and lotions are better than creams, since creams can trap moisture. Still, the best course is to avoid it. Here's how.

Sock it to 'em. When you take off your socks, rub one up and down in the webs between your toes, advises Dr. Basler. This helps keep feet desert-dry. Or you can use a hair dryer set on low to dry those trouble spots. And if you have a problem with sweating after your feet have been dried, you can roll on some antiperspirant after showering, he adds.

Be a shoe swapper. Try wearing different pairs of shoes as often as possible, says Dr. Basler. After a day's use, shoes are full of moisture and need at least a day to dry out. If you don't have many shoes, spray the pair you've worn with Lysol at the end of the day to help disinfect them and prevent athlete's foot.

Get cooking with baking soda. There are plenty of over-the-counter powders to prevent athlete's foot, but baking soda does essentially the same thing for a lot less money, says Dr. Levine. Just sprinkle it on daily to absorb excess moisture.

Ingrown Toenails

All it takes is a teeny bit of nail to cause big-time pain. Tight shoes can contribute to this problem by forcing the nail downward. If your nail is ingrown to the point that you're in constant agony, you may need a doctor to remove it. If not, here's how to keep nails trouble-free.

Cut nails straight across. The best way to cure an ingrown nail and prevent a new one from forming is to cut the nail straight across, not slightly curved or in a half-moon shape as most people do, says William Van Pelt, D.P.M., a Houston podiatrist and former president of the American Academy of Podiatric Sports Medicine. And don't cut it too short; it should be just over the crease of your nail fold. Be sure to soak your feet in warm water beforehand to make cutting easier.

Take your piggies to market. There are several over-the-counter products that can relieve pain by softening an ingrown nail and the skin around it. Dr. Levine recommends Dr. Scholl's ingrown toenail reliever and Outgro solution. Don't use these products if you have diabetes or circulation problems, however, because they contain strong acids that could be dangerous to people who have limited sensation in their feet.

GRAY HAIR

Showing Your True Colors

You roll out of bed, move slowly to the bathroom, and turn on the light. You lean toward the mirror for a close, close look. How many more gray hairs will there be today?

Besides wrinkles and sagging skin, few things shout "aging" to us louder than gray hair. While some of us love the look and wear it well, a whole lot of us don't. And there's a multi-million-dollar industry out there that caters to our need to keep our changing true colors a secret.

"If you're going gray, I guarantee that you're not happy about it," says Philip Kingsley, a hair-care specialist based in New York City. "I have seen tens of thousands of people over the years, and none of them wants gray hair. It can really make people feel old before their time."

Most of us have about 100,000 hairs on our heads. Before we go gray, every one of those hairs contains the pigment melanin, which gives hair its color. But for reasons that doctors don't understand, the pigment cells near the root of each hair start to shut down as we get older. So when a blond, brown, or red hair falls out, it's often replaced by a white one, although we call it gray because that's what it looks like in contrast to the hair that still has color.

If you're looking for someone to blame, start with Mom or Aunt Judith or great-grandpa Joe. "There's a very strong hereditary link with gray hair," says Diana Bihova, M.D., clinical assistant professor of dermatology at New York University Medical Center in New York City. "If your family went gray early, it's very likely that you will, too."

Whatever you do, though, don't chalk it up to stress. The stress of work, kids, and life in general won't give you gray hair, Dr. Bihova says.

The good news in all of this is that getting gray hair usually doesn't mean that there's anything physically wrong: It's not an indication that you're aging faster than friends who don't have a single gray strand yet. Studies show that people who go gray at an early age are usually not suffering from anything but a case of unwelcome family genetics.

The bad news is that graying is irreversible. That leaves you with two choices: You can accept it as an inescapable, even desirable, part of maturing, or you can put it on hold for a while by using some form of hair dye.

Let It Be

"Some people grow to be quite comfortable with gray hair," Kingsley says. "The most important point to remember about gray hair, or hair in general, is that you have to be comfortable with it. If it makes you feel wise or dignified, that's fine." If you decide to try the gray look, here's how to keep it looking great.

Crop it. Kingsley suggests keeping your hair cut short. "It's really simple," Kingsley says. "If you don't want gray hair or you're not sure about it, then short styles leave less gray to show."

Condition it. As time passes, your hair and scalp may get drier. To keep your gray looking healthy, Kingsley suggests using a conditioner each time you shampoo. And he suggests letting your hair air-dry once in a while instead of using a blow-dryer.

Color Choices

On the other hand, if you decide that you're not comfortable with silver locks, here are several options for using color effectively.

Bring on the highlights. Highlighting, in which scattered strands of hair are dyed, can subtly blend away some of the gray. Choose a color that's a couple of shades lighter than your natural hair. Lighter shades also help you avoid unsightly gray roots. When your hair grows out, the gray won't show as much.

Go all the way. The experts call this process color, and it means that all of your hair will be dyed one shade. If you opt for this, stay away from the darkest shades, which tend to make your hair look flat and unnatural. "Black colors don't really work well," Kingsley says. "All the hair is colored exactly the same, and you can instantly see that it's dyed."

There's also some question about whether dark hair dyes can cause cancer. Some studies have linked the use of such dyes to increased risk of bone cancer and lymphoma.

The bottom line? "There isn't one yet," says Sheila Hoar Zahm, Ph.D., an epidemiologist at the National Cancer Institute in Rockville, Maryland. "The risk of getting cancer from hair dye isn't as high as that of getting lung cancer from smoking. But we definitely need to study the relationship further."

Make it all or nothing. Kingsley says that you should be wary of progressive dyes that promise to slowly hide your gray hair. He says that these products can give your hair an unnatural, yellowish-green tint. They can also dry out your hair, making it unmanageable and brittle.

And once you start using them, it's hard to switch over to a regular dye. "That can turn your hair all sorts of colors that you would never want hair to be," Kingsley says.

Semipermanent dyes that wash out over several weeks offer somewhat better color but are not as good as permanent dyes. If you want to try a slow route to darker hair, Kingsley suggests doing it with increasingly darker permanent dyes.

HAIR LOSS

Winning over Thinning

So far, you've been able to hide it with certain haircuts or combing techniques, and it doesn't look like anybody has noticed yet. Still, it's getting harder and harder to deny that just like millions of other people, you're starting to lose your hair. Now you're worried sick, checking the mirror constantly—and feeling older by the minute.

Hair loss used to be considered a man's problem, since guys start balding as early as age 18. Only 12 percent of men are balding at age 25, but the figure jumps to 37 percent at age 35 and 45 percent at age 45. Two-thirds of all men are bald or balding by age 65. Women aren't spared either; at least 20 million American women are balding, and this can be even harder for them than it is for men.

"Hair is very much part of a woman's body image," says Dominic A. Brandy, M.D., medical director of Dominic A. Brandy, M.D., and Associates, a permanent hair restoration practice in Pittsburgh. "Losing it can cause a great deal of stress and, in some cases, can make women lose a certain amount of respect for themselves."

Not for Men Only

Heredity plays a role in as much as 85 percent of hair loss. If one or both of your parents or grandparents had thinning hair, you might, too, says Marty Sawaya, M.D., Ph.D., assistant professor of dermatology at the University of Florida Health Science Center in Gainesville.

Men first lose hair on the crown and at the hairline, while women are more likely to lose it evenly over the entire scalp. No one is quite sure what causes hair to stop growing. Whatever the cause, the sad truth is that short of drugs or hair transplants, there's really not much that you can do to stop your hair from thinning. Ken Hashimoto, M.D., professor of dermatology at Wayne State University School of Medicine in Detroit, stresses that miracle hair treatments—massages, topical creams, megavitamins, and the rest—do absolutely no good.

But don't give up just yet. Science still has a few options for you to try.

Pop some pills. The newest remedy for baldness in men is Propecia, a prescription drug recently approved by the Food and Drug Administration to prevent hair loss and increase hair growth. It is the first and only pill that's currently available to treat male pattern baldness. Propecia is a one-milligram formulation of finasteride, a substance that inhibits an enzyme called 5 alpha-reductase, which converts testosterone to dihydrotestosterone (DHT)—the male hormone that triggers male pattern baldness in men.

"Propecia both prevents the aging of hair and helps people keep the hair they have," says Peter Panagotacos, M.D., a dermatologist and expert in hair replacement in private practice in San Francisco. Dr. Panagotacos tells patients that they can expect to see results in four to six months.

What about side effects? In clinical studies, 2 percent of men did report impotence and a lessened desire for sex, but these effects disappeared in the 58 percent of men who continued treatment. Propecia is going to cost you about $45 per month and is only available by prescription. Check with your doctor about treatment and other possible side effects.

Regain it with Rogaine. A topical solution to baldness is the over-the-counter hair-restoring formula minoxidil lotion (Rogaine), which actually works to prevent hair loss or restore hair. "Minoxidil is like life support for an ailing follicle, whereas Propecia may tell the follicle not to get old in the first place," says Dr. Panagotacos.

Minoxidil comes in 2 and 5 percent strengths. The 5 percent lotion is for men only, as it may cause facial hair growth in women. The formula works by sparking withered or "miniaturized" hair follicles to return to their normal size and sprout wider, more youthful hair. Dr. Panagotacos suggests that you start with the 2 percent formula. "If you've used the 2 percent minoxidil," he says, "then the 5 percent may produce better results."

But minoxidil isn't perfect, he says. It works better at the top of the head than at the hairline and better on a small bald spot than on a big one. And while it can artificially stimulate hair regrowth in those with recent hair loss, it's not very good at restoring hair for men who have been bald a long time. Plus, you must use it every day, twice a day, for the rest of your life. Stop using it, and you'll lose the hair you've regained. Finally, some users experience some scalp itching, inflammation, dryness, or flaking, says Dr. Panagotacos.

Saving It with Surgery

If your problem is hereditary and there's no chance that your hair will bounce back to its youthful look by itself, you might want to consider hair replacement surgery. Years ago, hair transplants were easy to spot and often not worth the expense, but technology and technique have improved dramatically, Dr. Brandy says. And yes, women are having them done, even though the majority of patients are still men. There are several types of hair replacement procedures available, according to Dr. Brandy.

HAIR TRANSPLANTS. They've been around for about 35 years. The old practice involved moving large plugs of hair follicles (8 to 20 at a time) from the back of a patient's head, then embedding them in a balding area. This often resulted in uneven, unnatural hairlines.

Dr. Brandy says new micrografting surgical techniques allow doctors to transplant as few as one hair at a time. Dr. Brandy says this procedure is especially good for women, who usually don't have large bald spots to cover. The total cost can range from $3,500 to $10,000.

HAIR-LIFTS. These are more often used for men, since they are designed to cover large bald spots. The procedure involves cutting away bald scalp, then stretching hair-covered scalp from the sides and back of the head over the patient's crown. The procedure can cost between $3,500 and $5,000, Dr. Brandy says.

SCALP REDUCTION. This is a scaled-down version of the hair-lift. It involves removing smaller bald spots by stretching hair-covered scalp over the bald areas. The cost is about $2,500 to $3,000.

Another option is hair weaving, which is not a surgical procedure but a cosmetic treatment in which technicians splice natural or synthetic extensions to existing hair to make it look fuller. While it may be cheaper than surgery in the short run, Dr. Brandy says the extensions must be adjusted every four to six weeks as your hair grows.

Short Cuts to Thicker Hair

In addition to medical treatments, there are other ways to put body back into your thinning hair or prevent it from spoiling your overall look. Here's how.

Do the wave. The fastest way to hide thinning hair is with a curly perm, according to David Cannell, Ph.D., corporate vice president of technology with the Redken Product Laboratory in Canoga Park, California.

"With a wavy pattern, individual hairs push against each other," Dr. Cannell says. "The overall effect is that they push up and out, making your hair look fuller."

For men, keeping hair short can be helpful. Clipping it to a length of one-half to one inch will make it look neat and natural.

Get in condition. Avoid oily hair dressings and other products that advertise "creamy-rich" results. Dr. Cannell says these tend to weigh hair down and flatten it, which can make your hair look thin. He suggests trying a lighter, leave-in conditioner that may add a microscopic amount of thickness to individual hairs.

Give yourself a pat on the head. After showering, dry your hair carefully. Pat it lightly with a towel instead of rubbing.

Comb with care. Dr. Cannell advises using brushes and combs gently. Never brush your hair when it's wet (pulling on a tangle is always a no-no). Try using a comb with widely spaced teeth instead. And guys, forget the comb-over, says George Roberson, author of *Men's Hair*. You won't fool anyone by growing a foot-long piece of hair on the side of your head and plastering it over your bald spot.

Lighten up. Women should choose a new, lighter hair color. Shades that closely match your skin tone are best, Dr. Cannell says, since they blend with your scalp.

"The worst thing you can do is dye your hair jet-black," Dr. Cannell says. "That really shows your scalp, which is the last thing you want to do."

Keep your hands off. Drop nervous habits such as tugging on your hair or curling it with your fingers. You may be pulling on it more than you realize, since you're conscious of how it looks. "Even when a hair is ready to fall out, it will stick around for quite a while if you leave it be," Dr. Cannell explains. "The more you manipulate it, the faster it will go."

Try hair elsewhere. For men, a neat beard and mustache can draw people's eyes south, from your forehead to your face, says Roberson.

HEARING LOSS

Fending Off the Sounds of Silence

Kathy Peck loved head-banging music. As the bass player and lead singer in a punk rock band called The Contractions, she always figured the louder the music, the better.

But after the band got its big break as the opening act for Duran Duran at the Oakland Coliseum, Peck noticed that her hearing was fading fast. "After that show, I had ringing in my ears, and when I tried to talk with friends, I could see their lips move, but I couldn't hear any sound. I was basically deaf for days."

Soon afterward, testing revealed that she had a suffered a 40 percent hearing loss. Depressed, Peck worried about her career and wondered if Father Time was catching up with her, even though she was only in her early thirties.

But as Peck and other people are discovering, hearing loss in their thirties and forties is all too common. Overall, about 23 million Americans have significant hearing impairment, and almost 7 million of them are under age 45, according to the American Speech-Language-Hearing Association.

Some hearing loss is a natural part of aging, but the most common cause in adults under age 50 is excessive noise exposure, says Susan Rezen, Ph.D., professor of audiology at Worcester State College in Massachusetts and author of *Coping with Hearing Loss*. "The effects of noise exposure are long-term," she says. "They don't show up right away. But when people are continually exposed, their ears wear out faster, and the effects of aging show up earlier."

Protection Is the Key

Although most of us will suffer some hearing loss due to aging, you can keep your hearing sharp well into your golden years if you protect your ears from noise now. Here are some strategies.

Turn it down. You probably can't do much about traffic noise, jackhammers, and many other sources of excessive sound, but you can turn down the volume on your stereo, says Stephen Painton, Ph.D., an audiologist at the University of Oklahoma Health Sciences Center in Oklahoma City. Some sound systems can produce noise equal to that at the loudest rock concerts.

Here's a way to tell if your stereo is too loud. Turn it on, then walk outside your home and close the door. If you can hear the music, it's too loud. The same rule applies to your car radio. And if you use headphones or a personal stereo, the person standing next to you shouldn't be able to hear the sound.

If you have to shout, get out. If you have to raise your voice to be heard by someone standing a foot or two away from you, that's a clear warning that the noise level around you may be dangerous, and you should get away from it as soon as possible or wear ear protection, says John House, M.D., associate clinical professor of otolaryngology at the University of Southern California in Los Angeles.

Keep plugs handy. Get in the habit of carrying earplugs with you, says Debra Busacco, Ph.D., an audiologist and coordinator of the Lifelong Learning Institute at Gallaudet University in Washington, D.C. Most earplugs are small and can easily be carried in your purse or pocket. That way, she says, you'll be prepared for unexpected noise, such as an unusually loud movie. The foam rubber types are good because they are inexpensive and available over the counter at most drugstores, and they can be quickly rolled up and placed in your ears.

Look on the side of the box for the noise-reduction rating, which will tell you how many decibels of sound the earplugs will muffle, Dr. Painton says. Buy plugs that have a rating of at least 15, which means that they will reduce noise by 15 decibels and slash the chances that your hearing will be damaged.

If you want better protection, for about $80, an audiologist can design a pair of custom-made plugs that reduce noise by about 35 decibels, Dr. Busacco says.

Take time-outs. The longer you expose yourself to loud sounds without a break, the more likely you are to cause permanent damage to your hearing, even if you're wearing earplugs. So give your ears a 5- to 10-minute break from noise every 30 minutes, says Flash Gordon, M.D., a primary care physician in San Rafael, California. "If you give your ears an occasional break, they can rest and recover from the excessive work that loud noise makes them do."

Spread out the noise. Placing several loud appliances or power tools near each other can compound a noise problem. If your TV is in the same room as your dishwasher, for example, you might be tempted to turn up the TV volume when you do a load of dishes. Instead, move the television into a quieter room, says Lt. Col. Richard Danielson, Ph.D., supervisor of audiology in the Army Audiology and Speech Center at Walter Reed Army Medical Center in Washington, D.C.

Swab the deck, not your ears. Attempting to clean wax out of your ears does more harm than good, Dr. House says. Earwax is actually good for you, as it repels water and helps keep dust away from your sensitive eardrum. Sticking small objects into your ear pushes the wax farther into your ear and can cause infection. "The best thing to do about earwax inside the ear canal is to leave it alone," he says. If it becomes bothersome, see your physician or get an over-the-counter earwax removal kit that contains drops that will soften the wax and allow it to flow out naturally.

Don't puff. Smoking reduces blood flow to the ears and may interfere with the natural healing of small blood vessels that occurs after exposure to loud noise, Dr. House says. In a study of 2,348 workers exposed to noise at an aerospace factory, researchers at the University of Southern California School of Medicine found that smokers had greater hearing loss than nonsmokers. So if you smoke, quit.

Slash the java. Like nicotine, caffeine cuts blood flow to the ears, increasing your chances of hearing loss, Dr. House says. Drink no more than two eight-ounce cups of coffee or tea a day. If possible, drink decaffeinated brews.

Balance your diet. The same cholesterol-laden foods that are bad for your heart also endanger your ears, Dr. House says. They can reduce blood flow to the ears and gradually strangle your hearing. So cut the fat with a balanced daily diet that includes at least five servings of fruits and vegetables, six servings of breads and grains, and no more than one three-ounce serving of lean red meat, poultry, or fish.

Exercise. Walk, run, swim, or do any other aerobic exercise for 20 minutes a day, three times a week, Dr. House suggests. It will stimulate blood circulation, lower your blood pressure, and help keep your ears in peak condition.

Making the Best of It

The average person waits five to seven years after first noticing a hearing problem to seek help for it. If you suspect that you aren't hearing as well as you used to, see your doctor or a physician who specializes in diseases of the ear, nose, and throat.

Here's how to recognize if you have a hearing loss as well as some ways to cope with it.

Tune in to your turn signal. Sure, it's annoying when you drive down the road and realize that your turn signal has been on for miles, but it could also be a clue that you have a hearing problem. If you snap on your turn signal and can't hear the accompanying clicking sound in your car, it's time to get your hearing checked by an audiologist or doctor, Dr. Painton says.

Don't be shy about it. If you have difficulty hearing or understanding people, tell them, says Philip Zazove, M.D., assistant professor of family medicine at the University of Michigan Medical School in Ann Arbor, who has had profound hearing loss since birth. Simply saying, "I don't hear as well as I used to," "Could you repeat that?" and "Talk a little slower" can prevent a lot of misunderstandings, frustration, and anger, he says. If necessary, ask the person to repeat herself, or if you have trouble with a key word, have her write it on a piece of paper.

Do your homework. If you're attending an important business meeting or conference, get there early and try to nab a front-row seat facing the person who's likely to do most of the talking, Dr. Zazove says. Maintain eye contact with the speaker. Try to get a written summary of the topic or agenda so you'll be prepared for words or phrases that might come up. That way, if you do miss a few words, you'll have a better chance of filling them in accurately.

HIGH
BLOOD PRESSURE

The Silent Thief of Youth

Wrinkles we can see. Sore muscles we can feel. But there's a hidden aging problem out there, one that's far more dangerous than varicose veins, farsightedness, or gray hair. High blood pressure, also called hypertension, is directly linked to the deaths of more than 31,000 Americans each year, and it contributes to the deaths of untold thousands more. It can make us 12 times more likely to suffer strokes, 6 times more likely to suffer heart attacks, and 5 times more likely to die of congestive heart failure. It's also a major risk factor for kidney failure.

Yet, nearly half the people in this country with high blood pressure don't even know they have it. "There really aren't any noticeable outward signs. But if you have high blood pressure, it is doing damage," says Patrick Mulrow, M.D., chairman of the department of medicine at the Medical College of Ohio at Toledo and chairman of the American Heart Association's Council for High Blood Pressure Research.

In 90 to 95 percent of cases, Dr. Mulrow says, the exact cause of high blood pressure is unknown. But researchers have identified a number of factors that may increase your risk of developing high blood pressure. Family history is one. If several members of your immediate family have high blood pressure, you're more likely to develop it. African-Americans and members of other minority groups are at higher risk than whites. Obesity is another major factor. Studies show that 60 percent of people with high blood pressure are overweight. Psychological factors like job-related stress can also play a role. A study of 129 working adults found that people with high-status, high-pressure jobs showed significantly bigger increases in blood pressure during the workday than those with less-demanding jobs.

There's also a link between birth control pills and high blood pressure for some women, according to Dr. Mulrow. The newer low-dose oral contraceptives have greatly decreased the problem of elevated blood pressure, although smoking and taking the Pill will increase your chances of high blood pressure, he says.

Keeping It under Control

There are lots of prescription drugs that can help reduce high blood pressure. Diuretics flush excess fluids from the body. Beta-blockers reduce the heart rate and the heart's total output of blood. Vasodilators widen arteries and allow easier blood flow. Sympathetic nerve inhibitors also prevent blood vessels from constricting.

But drugs should be a last resort. They can cause fatigue and inhibit your sex life, among other side effects. The trick is to avoid high blood pressure in the first place, and the tips below will get you started. Even if you already have mild high blood pressure, these techniques could reduce your dependence on drugs and maybe even let you control things naturally.

Have it tested. There's only one way to know for sure if you have high blood pressure: Have your doctor check it. Once a year should be sufficient, unless your doctor orders more tests. It's a quick, painless procedure. The doctor or nurse puts an inflatable cuff around your arm and checks your pulse with a stethoscope. If you show a borderline high reading, the doctor may order several retests over a couple of weeks or months.

Be careful with the do-it-yourself blood pressure monitors in drugstores, grocery stores, and shopping malls, though. Dr. Mulrow warns that these machines aren't a substitute for an annual doctor's visit because some of them aren't well-calibrated and provide grossly inaccurate results. Too many external factors, such as whether you've been walking or are wearing a thick sleeve, also can interfere.

Lighten up. If you're overweight, even moderate weight loss may help lower your blood pressure, says Marvin Moser, M.D., clinical professor of medicine at Yale University School of Medicine and senior adviser to the National High Blood Pressure Education Program. In some cases, he says, weight loss of 10 to 15 pounds may be enough to lower slightly elevated blood pressure to normal and help you avoid medication.

A nationwide study of 162 overweight women, ages 30 to 54, showed how well weight loss can work. Over a 12-month period, the women on a weight-loss program lost an average of 6 pounds. Their systolic readings (the top number) fell an average of 3.7 points, while diastolic readings (the bottom number) fell 4.1 points. Another study of 362 overweight men, ages 30 to 54, showed that over a 12-month period, the men on a weight-loss program lost an average of 12 pounds; their systolic readings fell an average of 6 points, while diastolic readings fell 6.4 points.

Move it. Exercise, combined with a low-fat diet, is the best way to lose weight and keep your arteries clog-free. Research shows that people who don't exercise are 35 to 50 percent more likely to develop high blood pressure. And the American College of Sports Medicine says that regular aerobic training can reduce systolic and diastolic blood pressure by as much as 10 points.

You don't have to be a marathon runner to reap the benefits either. In fact, some studies have found that lower-intensity workouts such as walking are as good or better at lowering blood pressure than running or other heavy-duty aerobic activities. Many experts recommend working out at least three times a week for 20 minutes at a time.

Shake it off. The amount of sodium in the foods we eat is one of the biggest contributors to high blood pressure, experts say. Sodium makes us retain water, Dr. Mulrow says, which increases the volume of blood in our bodies and makes our hearts work harder to pump it.

Cut salt from your diet wherever you can. Most of us are eating about 2½ times more than we should. Research shows that three-fourths of all the salt we eat comes from processed foods such as cheese, soup, bread, baked goods, and snacks.

"You have to read labels," Dr. Mulrow says. Check for sodium content and shoot for a daily total of about 2,400 milligrams. When shopping, look for labels that say "low sodium." That means that they contain no more than 140 milligrams of sodium per serving. And spend some extra time in the produce aisle. Almost every fruit and vegetable is naturally low in sodium.

Be careful when you eat out, too. You'll be surprised how fast sodium can add up. A hamburger from your favorite fast-food restaurant, for instance, may give you almost half a day's quota.

Pile on the potassium. Studies have shown that a daily intake of 3,500 milligrams of potassium can help counteract sodium and keep blood volume—and blood pressure—down. And it's easy to get enough. A baked potato packs 838 milligrams of potassium all by itself, and one cup of spinach has 800 milligrams. Other potassium-packed foods include bananas, orange juice, corn, cabbage, and broccoli. Check with your doctor before taking potassium supplements, though, as too much may aggravate kidney problems.

Meet your magnesium needs. Researchers seem to have found a link between low magnesium intake and high blood pressure. But just how much magnesium you need to combat high blood pressure remains unclear. For now, your best bet is to get the Daily Value of about 400 milligrams, says Robert DiBianco, M.D., director of cardiology research at the Washington Adventist Hospital in Takoma Park, Maryland.

Unfortunately, America's intake of magnesium has been dropping for a century, since we started processing foods and robbing them of their trace elements. Good sources of magnesium include nuts, spinach, lima beans, peas, and seafood. But don't overdo it by taking supplements; Dr. Mulrow says too much magnesium can give you a nasty case of diarrhea.

Fill up with fiber. A Swedish study of 32 people with mild high blood pressure found that taking a seven-gram tablet of fiber each day helps lower diastolic blood pressure by five points. No one is sure why; perhaps it's due to weight loss that occurs because fiber makes people feel fuller and eat less or because they eat less sodium. Whatever the reason, seven extra grams of fiber is easy to find. There's almost that much in a bowl of high-fiber cereal.

Drink in moderation. "A little alcohol isn't going to hurt," Dr. Mulrow says. "But drinking every day, and drinking to excess, could mean trouble." For women fighting high blood pressure, the equivalent of three ounces of alcohol a week seems to be about the limit. A 12-year study of 1,643 women, with an average age of 47, showed that both systolic and diastolic pressure readings begin to rise steadily after that point. That means three beers, three glasses of wine, or three cocktails containing hard liquor.

Stop smoking. Smoking markedly increases your risk of developing a stroke or blood vessel damage from high blood pressure, says Dr. Mulrow. When you smoke, it encourages your body to deposit cholesterol within your coronary arteries. This decreases the size of your vessels and forces your heart to work harder. "Anyone with high blood pressure should stop smoking immediately," he advises.

IMPOTENCE

Living Well Shrinks Your Risk

The woman of your dreams stands before you in a seductive red teddy. She leans over, kisses you passionately, and beckons you toward the bedroom. Your pulse quickens, your breathing speeds up, and all systems are go. But then, suddenly, your rocket launcher loses power.

Uh, oh. You've heard that it happens to every guy at one time or another, so you try to shrug it off. But you can't, and all of a sudden getting an erection seems more difficult than hauling a 1,000-pound piano up three flights of stairs.

Preserving Potency

When you're in your twenties, you never think twice about getting an erection. By the time you creep toward 40, your sexual responses are less predictable . But in reality, few men in their thirties and forties are impotent, and there are many things that you can do to make sure that you won't ever be. If you are impotent, in many cases it can be cured. Here are few ways to keep your private parts in good working order.

Cut out the smoke signals. Smoking accelerates the formation of blockages in the heart's arteries, and there's every reason to believe that it does the same to the vessels that supply blood to the penis. In fact, smoking is now considered a major factor in erection problems, with the first signs of harm appearing by age 40. So if you smoke, quit, says Roger Crenshaw, M.D., a psychiatrist and sex therapist in private practice in La Jolla, California.

Run, don't walk, to the gym. The fitter you are, the more sex you'll have, and the better it will be, says a study published in the *Archives of Sexual Behavior*. In the study, conducted at the University of California, San Diego, 78 healthy but inactive men began aerobic exercise three to five days a week for an hour each time. Another group simply walked at a moderate pace three to five days a week. During the study, each man kept a diary of sexual activity. The results showed that the sex lives of the aerobic exercisers significantly improved, while the sex lives of the walkers changed very little.

It doesn't matter which type of aerobic exercise you choose, as long as you do it a minimum of three times each week and stick with it for at least 20 minutes per session. Running, swimming, and rowing are good choices, Dr. Crenshaw says.

Nix the fat. When it comes to diet, the bottom line is limiting your fat intake. Again, logic says that what's good for the arteries supplying blood flow to the heart will also be good for those supplying blood to the penis.

A high-potency diet should be low in fat, with about 20 percent of its calories from fat, says Joseph Khoury, M.D., a urologist in private practice in Bethesda, Maryland. If you eat 2,500 calories a day, that would be about 50 grams of fat. To get started in the right direction, read food labels, look for low-fat and nonfat products, avoid fried foods, switch to skim milk, and eat at least five half-cup servings of fruits and vegetables every day, along with one three-ounce serving (about the size of a deck of cards) of fish, poultry, or lean red meat.

Trim your waistline. Excess pounds can actually make important inches of the penis disappear. Informal studies of overweight men by John Mulcahy, M.D., professor of urology at the Indiana University Medical Center in Indianapolis, show that—up to a point—an overweight man will regain one inch of his penis for every 35 pounds of weight lost. Not a bad incentive for someone who's really heavy. But more practically, keeping your weight down will reduce the risk of high blood pressure and diabetes, both of which impair the ability to have an erection.

Watch your drug use. Hundreds of drugs, including diuretics, high blood pressure medications, and some antidepressants and antipsychotics, can cause impotence as a side effect. Ask your doctor or pharmacist if medication could be causing your problem.

Go light on the booze. Alcohol is a depressant that slows down reflexes, including sexual ones. Besides impairing immediate performance, alcohol, when consumed excessively for too long, can have a direct effect on the testicles, decreasing production of the male hormone testosterone and upsetting the delicate balance of hormones and brain chemicals that are required to get an erection. Limit yourself to two beers or glasses of wine a day, suggests Saul Rosenthal, M.D., director of the Sexual Therapy Clinic of San Antonio in Texas and author of *Sex over 40*. If you're having sexual difficulty, stop drinking for three months to see if that helps, he advises.

Be on guard. Penile fracture is an all-too-common cause of impotence, says Irwin Goldstein, M.D., professor of urology at Boston University School of Medicine. "Fracturing the penis breaks the fibrous lining that contains the pressure that allows you to have an erection. It literally cracks like the wall of a tire that goes over a curb too fast," he says. The most vulnerable position is when the woman is on top, because the penis can slip out of her vagina and she can slam her pelvis down on it. Abnormal bending during sex, bicycling accidents, and blows to the crotch can also damage the penis and testicles.

Look at your relationship. Often, your sexual relationship reflects what is going on with your partner outside of bed. "If your relationship with the woman is unhealthy, impotence could be your body's way of giving you an early warning that something is wrong, and you should try to interpret your body's signals in order to understand the meaning of your response," says Herb Goldberg, Ph.D., a clinical psychologist in Los Angeles and author of *The Inner Male*.

Leave your anger at the door. Anger can inhibit sexual arousal, says Domeena Renshaw, M.D., director of the Sexual Dysfunction Clinic at Loyola University of Chicago Stritch School of Medicine. A classic example of this is a fellow who had a vicious argument with his ex-wife over an upcoming weekend visit with his three-year-old son. The conversation stayed in his mind the entire evening.

"My girlfriend was dressed to kill, and she was in the mood," he says. "But all I could think about was how to strangle my ex-wife. Nothing was happening below the belt."

Talk about your anger and frustration with your partner outside the bedroom. Letting it fester will only put a clamp on your erections.

Get real. There's no point in trying to compete with your 20-year-old self. You are bound to have a bit less spontaneity in your sex life than you had then, if only because you have more on your mind, greater responsibilities, richer interests, a fuller schedule, and more stress, says Jack Jaffe, M.D., director of the Potency Recovery Center in Van Nuys, California. The way to avoid psychological problems that could interfere with your performance is not to wait for the magic moment. "You have to make it happen," he says. "That may mean setting a date, sitting down to discuss what your needs are, whatever it takes."

MENOPAUSAL CHANGES

They're Bound to Happen

You had an unsettling conversation with your best friend the other day, and you still can't get it out of your mind.

"I've noticed some changes in my body lately," she said, "and I can't help wondering if I'm starting."

"Starting what?" you asked, half distracted by thoughts of your upcoming vacation.

"Menopause."

Menopause! That sure caught your attention. Your friend—who's only a few years older than you—was actually experiencing something that neither of you thought you had to worry about yet. Isn't it too soon? you wondered. You're both under 50, and you always felt that menopause was meant for your mother, your great-aunt, and other, well, *older* women.

For most women, menopause is a landmark of aging, says Ellen Klutznick, Psy.D., a psychologist in San Francisco who specializes in women's issues. And how women respond to it varies widely. Technically, a woman is considered to be menopausal when she has not menstruated for a year. The average age for menopause in the United States is 51, although women can go through it earlier. For several years prior to actual menopause—a stage called perimenopause—women can experience a whole range of physical changes, including hot flashes, night sweats, sleep difficulties, vaginal dryness, skin changes, hair loss, mood swings, depression, and weight gain. All of these symptoms as well as the actual cessation of periods are caused by a decrease in levels of the female hormone estrogen. The level of estrogen dips even further after menopause, and that decline can increase the risk of osteoporosis (brittle-bone disease) as well as heart disease.

Making It Manageable

Unfortunately, you can't avoid menopause. But there are some things that you can do now, before you get there, that can make the whole experience a little easier. Menopause doesn't have to be a trying time, and it doesn't have to make you look and feel older. Here's what experts recommend.

Get a move on it. Exercise is one of the best things women can do ahead of time in order to fare better during their menopausal years, says Brian Walsh, M.D., director of the Menopause Clinic at Brigham and Women's Hospital in Boston. Exercise places stress on bone, increasing its density and strength. Since women's bones lose density after menopause—at the rate of 4 to 6 percent in the first four to five years—the stronger they are to start off with, the better. Weight-bearing activities such as walking and running are best, experts say. Exercise also helps keep cholesterol levels down, thus offering protection against heart disease.

Eat right. Start eating a nutritious diet low in saturated fat, says Dr. Walsh. This will help reduce cholesterol and the risk of heart disease, he says, both of which go up after menopause. Experts recommend that you keep your fat intake at 25 percent or less of the total calories you consume.

Quit smoking. If you stop smoking at a younger age, it can help you experience a gentler menopause, says Dr. Walsh. Smokers are more likely than nonsmokers to have menopausal symptoms, he says. Smoking can also cause you to experience menopause earlier, experts say. They think it's because nicotine may somehow contribute to the drop in estrogen. Smokers also have a tendency toward lower bone mass, putting them at greater risk for osteoporosis.

Get your calcium now. After age 35, women lose 1 percent of their bone mass per year, so be sure to consume enough calcium. The Daily Value for calcium is 1,000 milligrams, but some experts suggest 1,500 milligrams for postmenopausal women who are not taking hormone replacement therapy and for all women over 65.

Unfortunately, most women consume only about 500 milligrams a day through diet. You can come closer to the protective amounts by adding low-fat dairy products, canned fish such as salmon (with the bones), and soy foods such as tofu to your daily diet.

Get support. "The most valuable thing is gathering together with other women," says Joan Borton, a licensed mental health counselor in private practice in Rockport, Massachusetts, and author of *Drawing from the Women's Well: Reflections on the Life Passage of Menopause.* By talking with other women, either one-on-one or in support groups, you can learn about various symptoms and gather information about doctors and health-care professionals to whom other women go and whom they like and recommend, she says.

"Talking with other women and sharing experiences helps women feel supported and not so isolated," agrees Dr. Klutznick. One option is to join a support group. To find out about groups in your area, call a local hospital or talk to other women.

Find the right doctor. Menopause will bring lots of physical changes and lots of questions, particularly about hormone replacement therapy (HRT). HRT is recommended to help replace missing estrogen and keep bones strong, but it is also controversial, mainly because it may increase your risk of certain cancers. "The key is to get a doctor who will work with you—one who will honor your decision," says Borton. Ask your friends about their doctors. And don't be afraid to shop around until you find a doctor you like.

Look for a mentor. Find a woman 10 to 15 years older than you who has been through menopause and whom you admire and respect, says Borton. "Spend time with older women, exploring with them what it is that holds meaning in their lives," she says. "Numbers of us feel that doing this has helped us cross the threshold into seeing ourselves as older women and embracing it in a way that feels really wonderful." In addition, look for older women in the public eye whom you can follow and learn from, she says.

Stay lubricated. The decrease in estrogen at menopause can cause vaginal dryness. The elasticity and size of the vagina change, and the walls become thinner and lose their ability to become moist. This can make sex painful or even undesirable, says Dr. Klutznick. Surveys indicate that this happens in 8 to 25 percent of postmenopausal women. While premenopausal women can generally lubricate in 6 to 20 seconds when aroused, it can take one to three minutes for a postmenopausal woman.

Water-based vaginal lubricants such as K-Y Jelly, Replens, and Astroglide, which are available over the counter, are helpful in replacing natural lubrication, says Dr. Klutznick. Steer clear of oil-based lubricants such as petroleum jelly, though, as studies indicate that they don't dissolve as easily in the vagina and can therefore trigger vaginal infections. HRT can also help alleviate dryness, she says.

Stay sexually active. Studies indicate that women who stay sexually active experience fewer vaginal changes than those who don't. Sexual activity promotes circulation in the vaginal area, which helps it stay moist. For women without partners, masturbation helps to promote circulation and moistness in the vagina, Dr. Klutznick says.

Keep it cool. The hot flashes that many women experience during menopause can range from warmth to burning heat that causes flushing and sweating. Experts don't completely understand what causes hot flashes, but they think that the decline in estrogen somehow upsets the body's internal thermometer. It can help to dress in layers and to keep the environment cool, experts say. Some women suck on ice cubes and drink cold liquids or visualize themselves walking in the snow or swimming in a clear lake. Hot liquids and spicy foods can trigger hot flashes, so keep those to a minimum.

OSTEOPOROSIS

Strengthening Your Support System

Your bones seem like steel girders—strong and permanent, a structure you can depend on. But for 1 in every 4 women and 1 in every 10 men, the girders weaken and wear away, eroding the skeletal structure.

The cause is osteoporosis, a disease of thinning bones, fractured hips, and hunched spines. It is a disease of aging that you can prevent—if you start today.

You can't stop your bones from thinning, as bone loss over time is normal. But if you have osteoporosis, the loss is a lot more rapid than usual, and your bones can become so brittle and fragile that they break when you step off a curb or bump a hip on the edge of a table. In fact, the bones in your spine—the vertebrae—can even break under your own weight.

Are You a Candidate?

If your mother or father has osteoporosis, you may also be prone to these frightening fractures, says Clifford Rosen, M.D., director of the Maine Center for Osteoporosis Research and Education in Bangor. "Up to 70 percent of your peak bone mass, which you reach in your twenties, is determined by heredity," he says.

One of the biggest causes of osteoporosis, however, is too little calcium in your diet. Although estimates of how many people are short on this basic bone-building nutrient vary from 10 to 25 percent, experts agree that calcium deficiency is extremely common. Vitamin D is another nutrient that's vital to bone health because it aids in the absorption of calcium. If you're not getting enough vitamin D, your body won't be able to take advantage of even generous amounts of calcium.

Other factors that contribute to osteoporosis are smoking and heavy drinking, experts say. Certain prescription medicines may also erode bone strength, particularly if taken for many years or in extremely high doses.

Although all doctors don't agree that everyone should be tested for osteoporosis, Dr. Rosen recommends that you play it safe and get a bone-density measurement of your hip and spine when you are between the ages of 45 and 55, when thinning bone is first detectable. The best test is called dual energy x-ray absorptiometry, or DEXA, and costs about $100 to $250. If a DEXA machine is not available in your community, your doctor can assess your bone health with a computerized axial tomography (CAT) scan instead.

Doctors agree that people at greatest risk for the disease—those with family histories of osteoporosis or personal histories of smoking or heavy drinking—should be tested before age 45.

Healthy Habits for Life and Limb

If your test shows a higher-than-normal level of bone loss, don't despair—you don't have to sit back and surrender to osteoporosis. You can minimize your risks and take definite steps to build stronger bones. What matters most is that you start now. Here are the best ways to strengthen your skeleton.

Pump up your calcium. Calcium is to your bones what air is to your lungs—the element they need to be healthy. Ninety-nine percent of the calcium in your diet goes straight to your bones. If you don't get enough calcium, you can't make enough bone—it's as simple as that.

Although the Daily Value for most people is 1,000 milligrams a day, you need more calcium in adolescence and after menopause, Dr. Rosen says. Postmenopausal women who are not taking estrogen and all women over 65 should get 1,500 milligrams. Although food is the best way to get calcium, what matters most is that you take in the recommended amount, he says. If you get that much through food, fine; if you use a combination of food and calcium supplements to meet your quota, that's also fine. Just make sure the numbers add up.

Ounce for ounce, milk and milk products are the best sources of dietary calcium. One eight-ounce serving of nonfat yogurt provides about 450 milligrams, and a cup of skim milk offers more than 300 milligrams. Many other foods contain calcium, but it isn't as easily absorbed from these foods as it is from dairy products.

Don't forget the D. Bones don't absorb calcium unless they have plenty of vitamin D, says Michael F. Holick, M.D., Ph.D., director of the Vitamin D, Skin, and Bone Research Laboratory at Boston University Medical Center. Without vitamin D, your body absorbs about 10 percent of the calcium it takes in; with vitamin D, it can absorb 80 to 90 percent. "Vitamin D tells the small intestine, 'Here comes the calcium. Open up and let it in,'" he explains. The Daily Value for vitamin D is 400 international units—easily found in fortified foods such as milk, breads, and cereals.

Besides getting some of your daily vitamin D through food, your body can make it from sunshine, which triggers a vitamin D manufacturing process in your skin. Exposure to bright sunshine for 5 to 15 minutes every day, before you apply sunscreen, will supply your needs, says Dr. Rosen. If you live north of New York City, however, you can't depend on the sun. In that case, you'll need to be sure you're getting enough vitamin D from dietary sources. (If you're getting plenty in your diet, you won't need time in the sun at all.)

Review your medication. Certain medications—thyroid medications; anti-inflammatory steroids such as hydrocortisone (Locoid), cortisone (Cortone Acetate), and prednisone (Key-Pred 50); anticonvulsants such as phenytoin (Dilantin); depressants such as phenobarbital (Barbita); and the diuretic furosemide (Lasix)—can cause osteoporosis, particularly when they're taken regularly in high doses over a number of years. Thyroid medications in normal doses should pose no problem, however, says Dr. Rosen, and the risk from diuretics can be offset by taking additional calcium. The most serious osteoporosis risk is from steroids, he advises. If you require long-term steroid medication, he continues, your doctor may recommend additional anti-osteoporosis medication such as calcitonin (Cibacalcin) or hormone replacement therapy in addition to calcium and vitamin D supplements.

Keep 'em dry and healthy. "Alcohol actually poisons the cells that build bone," says Susan Allen, M.D., Ph.D., assistant professor of internal medicine at the University of Missouri at Columbia School of Medicine. A beer or a glass of wine now and then probably won't cause you much harm. But avoid drinking to excess, she says—more than two to three drinks a day.

Grin and bear it. To strengthen bones, you need activities in which you're putting weight on them, Dr. Allen says. Weight-bearing exercises include brisk walking, jogging, and dancing, which actually stimulate bone cells to build more bone, particularly in your back and hips, where you need it most.

"Basically, you can count on any exercise that makes heavy use of gravity," says Dr. Rosen. "Swimming doesn't, for example, but most aerobics classes and tennis do."

Pumping iron is also an ideal way to build bone strength because it increases the weight of gravity on your bones. Any lifting done in a standing position is particularly helpful for the spine and hips. If you've never used weights before, be sure to get your doctor's clearance and a trainer's advice on the safest routine.

Do it regularly. Once you've found the weight-bearing exercises you like, keep at them for 30 minutes to one hour, three to four times a week, Dr. Allen says.

Concentrate on the back and hips. If you're exercising for weight loss and muscle tone, you're probably doing something for your upper body, and that's good. But remember, says Dr. Allen, the bones that are most vulnerable to osteoporosis are the hips and the spinal vertebrae in the mid to lower back. Walking, jogging, and aerobic dancing are particularly helpful for these areas, she says.

Don't puff. Smoking lowers estrogen levels, says Barbara S. Levine, Ph.D., associate clinical professor of nutrition in medicine and director of the Calcium Information Center at Cornell University Medical College in New York City. And lower estrogen, she says, means less protection against bone loss for women.

For male smokers, the risk of osteoporosis doubles, says Catherine Niewoehner, M.D., associate professor of medicine at the University of Minnesota in Minneapolis. Why? Smokers tend to be thinner, and thinner people are at greater risk for osteoporosis, she says. Researchers also theorize that the hormone testosterone may protect men from osteoporosis just as estrogen protects women and that male smokers lose more testosterone as they age than nonsmokers do. So do your bones a favor and give up the weed. If you need help, talk to your doctor.

Consider hormone replacement therapy. If you're a woman, that is. For some women past menopause, hormone replacement therapy can thicken bones. Ask your doctor whether you're a candidate for it.

OVERWEIGHT

Getting Yourself Down to Size

Everyone knows that you gain weight as you get older, right? Women get thunder thighs, and men get potbellies. It happened to your parents, and now that you're on the far side of 30, it's starting to creep up on you. And you don't like it one bit.

Being overweight is a burden on body and soul. You feel that you've lost your youth and vitality. And you've opened yourself up to ailments of aging such as heart disease, high blood pressure, diabetes, arthritis, and high cholesterol—not to mention the backaches and other pains caused by carrying around more than you should.

What can you do about it? Well, you could put yourself on a crash diet. But that probably won't get you anything but frustration. "Diets just don't work," says Janet Polivy, Ph.D., professor of psychology at the University of Toronto Faculty of Medicine. "Diets become popular because they work for a week or two and everyone says, 'You gotta try it.' Well, speak to those people in a year or two, and you'll find they've failed." When you fall for one of those speedy five-pounds-a-week programs, you lose it, all right—but you lose pounds of fluid, not fat. And as soon as you abandon the diet, the weight comes right back on.

Getting Started

For successful weight loss, before you get to the physical side of things, you need to lay down the mental and emotional groundwork. Here are the basics.

Make a long-term commitment. The key to healthy and successful weight loss at any age, experts say, is to make the changes gradually. Losing no more than one-half pound a week is ideal, says George Blackburn, M.D., Ph.D., chief of the Nutrition/Metabolism Laboratory at Beth Israel Deaconess Medical Center in Boston. So aim to attain a healthy weight a year from now, not next week, he says.

Surround yourself with support. A good support system is a key to successful weight loss, says John Foreyt, Ph.D., director of the Nutrition Research Clinic at Baylor College of Medicine in Houston. Ask your family and friends to cheer you on. Maybe they could join you in eating low-fat, healthful meals.

Pay attention to your emotional needs. Sometimes you can confuse hunger with other feelings, especially if you're feeling depressed or stressed or just responding to a luscious photo spread in a gourmet food magazine. If it's not your stomach talking, you need to figure out what kinds of emotions or discomforts are triggering your urge for food, Dr. Foreyt says. Then develop a problem-solving approach. "How can you answer that need without eating? Walk around the block, call a friend, meditate, take a bath, brush your teeth, or gargle with mouthwash," he says. "This breaks the chain and develops an alternate behavior pattern."

Losing Weight with Good Eatin'

The latest nutrition research shows that there really is a whole new way to lose weight—without dieting and without hunger. You may be surprised to find that the most crucial changes don't require that you eat less—just differently. Here's how.

Forgo excess fat. Dietary fat makes us gain weight because it's stored in the body far more easily than either carbohydrates or protein, says Peter D. Vash, M.D., assistant clinical professor of medicine at the University of California, Los Angeles. Fat also burns off very slowly and is more likely to be left over—on you. Start by cutting fat in the obvious places: Eat fewer fatty meats, fried foods, high-fat dairy products, and desserts. Also beware of salads slathered in oil or other fatty dressings. It's recommended that you keep your calories from fat to 25 percent or less of your daily total.

Drown it. "Drinking generous amounts of water is overwhelmingly the number one way to reduce appetite," says Dr. Blackburn. Water keeps your stomach feeling fuller, obviously, but it also may satisfy cravings since many people think they're having food cravings when they're actually thirsty, he says. So aim for eight cups of fluids daily, sipping a half-cup at a time through the day.

Count on carbs. When you replace the excess fat calories you've been eating with foods such as carbohydrates, you can actually eat more and still lose pounds. In one study at the University of Illinois at Chicago, people on moderately high fat diets were told to maintain their weights for 20 weeks while switching to low-fat, high-carbohydrate diets. They ate all they wanted and still lost more than 11 percent of their body fat and 2 percent of their weight. So enjoy plenty of carbohydrate-rich pasta (without fatty sauces), low-fat cereals, breads, beans, crunchy fresh vegetables, and fruits to fill you up while you're losing weight.

Allow a few splurges. If you feel that all you're saying to yourself about food is no-no-no, you may eventually let slips turn into a downhill slide, says Susan Kayman, R.D., Dr.P.H., a dietitian and consultant with the Kaiser Permanente Medical Group in Oakland, California. That's why she advocates following the 80/20 rule. If you eat low-fat 80 percent of the time, then when you're dining with friends, out on the town, or over at the in-laws, enjoy an occasional higher-fat treat without beating yourself up about it.

Break up the deadly duo. That's fats and sweets. When the body gets a jolt of sugar, it releases lots of insulin in response. Because insulin is a storage-prone hormone, it opens up fat cells, preparing them for fat storage. So when you eat sugar, keep your fat intake low. Also, soothe your sweet tooth with juicy fresh fruit or a bowl of low-fat sugared cereal instead of doughnuts and candy bars.

Eat often. Some researchers support the idea of grazing—eating numerous small meals throughout the day instead of three larger meals—to control appetite and prevent bingeing. "But you cannot graze on M&M's, potato chips, and Häagen-Dazs," says James Kenney, R.D., Ph.D., a nutrition research specialist at the Pritikin Longevity Center in Santa Monica, California. "But if you graze on low-fat, high-fiber foods that aren't packed with calories, such as carrots, apples, peaches, oranges, and red peppers, you'll keep your appetite down."

Ride out a craving. When the urge strikes for a chocolate eclair, don't confuse the craving with a command, says Linda Crawford, an eating behavior specialist in Ludlow, Vermont. Although many people think that cravings keep getting stronger until they're irresistible, research shows that food cravings actually start and escalate, then peak and subside. Distract yourself with a walk or something else incompatible with eating, Crawford says, and ride out the craving. "Just as with surfing," she says, "the more you practice riding a craving wave, the easier it becomes."

A Weight-Loss Workout

Adopting a healthier diet will help you lose weight, but you'll acquire a firmer figure faster—and keep it—if you combine your healthy new eating habits with exercise.

If you're unaccustomed to exercising, see your doctor before you get started. After you have the okay, you'll be ready. Here are some tips to get you going.

Keep it up. "The best predictor of long-term weight management is regular aerobic activity, which boosts your heart rate," says Dr. Foreyt. "Brisk walking is a great choice because it's very easy for most people to do on a regular basis. But the effectiveness of any aerobic activity for weight control has been proven repeatedly." Any kind of daily exercise helps. Thirty minutes of aerobic exercise burns flab and tones muscles—as long as you do it regularly.

Burn by building. Aerobic exercise should always be part of your weight-loss plan, but when you add resistance training such as weight lifting, you'll keep your weight down because of "hungry" muscles. "Muscle tissue needs more calories," says Janet Walberg-Rankin, Ph.D., associate professor of exercise science at Virginia Polytechnic Institute and State University in Blacksburg. "So if you increase muscle mass while you lose fat, you boost your ability to burn fuel."

To really work your muscles for weight loss, your best bet is to go to a gym and ask a trainer to show you how to circuit-train. You use a series of different weight machines to press weights against muscles in the neck, arms, chest, and legs. You can accomplish the same thing by working with free weights at home, says Dr. Foreyt. "Putting your muscles against something that doesn't yield—that's resistance."

PROSTATE PROBLEMS

Corralling the Male Menace

Lately, your urinary tract is acting like a worka-holic. It wakes you up in the middle of the night, interrupts your lunch, and yanks you out of important meetings, sending you scurrying to the bathroom. But even though you're in the men's room a lot these days, you never feel that you've finished what you went there to do.

You could blame your bladder, but in all probability, your prostate is the problem.

The prostate, a small gland about the size of a walnut, is wrapped around the urethra, the tube that drains the bladder. The prostate se-cretes the fluid and enzyme mixture that sperm require for good health and mobility. As you get older, the mild-mannered prostate can grad-ually turn into the gland from hell, becoming vulnerable to infection and disease—including cancer—and often swelling to the point where it interferes with urination.

Virtually every guy will have a prostate problem in his lifetime. Be-sides being a major nuisance, it's also the clarion call that youth is on the wane.

No, you don't need an exorcist to rid yourself of these woes, but you should see your doctor since the symptoms of minor prostate ail-ments are similar to those of serious disease. Those symptoms include frequent urination, blood in the urine, trouble starting the flow, weak flow, and a feeling that even when you're done, you're not quite finished. Let's take a look at the three most common problems.

BENIGN PROSTATIC HYPERPLASIA (BPH). As a man approaches his midforties, his prostate typically begins to swell. In some cases, it can grow to the size of a grapefruit and pinch off urine flow through the urethra, says Thomas Stanisic, M.D., a urologist in private practice in Ashland, Kentucky. The condition is BPH, and it is the most common prostate problem. It affects up to 15 percent of men over age 40 and 60 percent of men over 50.

PROSTATITIS. If you're only 35, however, and have difficult or frequent urination, it could be an infection known as bacterial prostatitis.

Bacterial prostatitis can affect men of all ages. It's usually caused by the spread of infection in the bladder or urethra. Although doctors aren't sure how the infection enters the urinary tract, some suspect that an obstruction in the urethra or unprotected anal sex increases the risk. Besides urination problems, the symptoms can include lower abdominal or back pain, discomfort in the testicles, and fever.

PROSTATE CANCER. Prostate cancer is the most common cancer among men over age 50 and the second leading killer among cancers in men in the United States. More than half of all men over 70 have it, says Dr. Stanisic.

It is usually curable if detected early, but often this cancer grows silently within the gland without any symptoms until it has spread to the surrounding bone and tissue. That's why it's important for men over age 50 to get a digital rectal exam that lets a doctor feel for lumps on the prostate and a prostate-specific antigen blood test that detects a protein that seeps out of the prostate when there is a tumor present.

If cancer is discovered, treatment will depend on the size of the tumor, how fast it is growing, and whether the disease has spread beyond the prostate. Treatments include radiation, surgical removal of the prostate, and hormone therapy to reduce testosterone levels.

Taming the Wild Prostate

As we said earlier, most men will experience one or more of these problems as they get older. But some doctors believe that you can reduce the possibility and impact of these diseases with a few dietary and lifestyle changes. Here's how.

Ejaculate regularly. Doing so may keep prostatic ducts from getting clogged and backed up. "It can only help," says Kenneth Goldberg, M.D., founder and director of the Male Health Center in Dallas.

Lower your cholesterol. Cholesterol is converted to testosterone in the body. It has been observed that enlarged prostate tissue is very high in cholesterol. Some doctors claim an improvement in symptoms, if not in prostate size, by getting patients to lower their total blood cholesterol levels to 200 mg/dl (milligrams of cholesterol per deciliter of blood) or less, as recommended by the American Heart Association.

Drop the fat. Avoid foods laden with fat, such as red meats, dairy products, and fried foods, Dr. Goldberg says. Limit yourself to one three-ounce serving of meat, fish, or poultry a day.

Eat more vegetables. Male hormone levels drop with a vegetarian diet, and that may explain why BPH is rarer in cultures whose diets are largely vegetarian, Dr. Goldberg says.

Get enough zinc. Men with prostate ailments tend to have low concentrations of zinc in their bodies, says Paul M. Block, M.D., a urologist in private practice in Phoenix. The Daily Value is 15 milligrams. Taking zinc supplements or eating foods rich in zinc, including herring and steamed oysters, can help. Oatmeal, wheat bran, milk, peas, and nuts also contain the mineral.

Limit spicy foods and alcohol. Both of these may increase bladder irritability, particularly if you have BPH, Dr. Block says. Alcohol can be especially tough since it's a central nervous system depressant that reduces muscle tone throughout the body, including in the bladder, causing it to retain urine.

Get your exercise. There's no prostate-specific workout, although drinking water, voiding on demand, and regular sexual relations help. But you should know that many physicians have observed that men in good shape are less likely to have prostate trouble than their sedentary brothers.

Don't hold it in. If you need to urinate frequently, logic may tell you to train your bladder by waiting as long as you can. Logic has been wrong before, and it's wrong here. "You may actually harm yourself by waiting too long," says Patrick C. Walsh, M.D., professor and chairman of urology at Johns Hopkins University in Baltimore. "When urine backs up too far, it can damage the kidneys." Urinate as soon as you feel the need.

Avoid drinking after dark. Forgo liquids after 6:00 or 7:00 P.M. if your sleep has been interrupted frequently (say, two or more times a night) by the urge to urinate, Dr. Block suggests. Day and night, limit drinks containing caffeine, as they make you urinate more and increase irritability of the bladder, causing it to feel full even when it isn't.

Soak it. Sit in a warm bath for 20 minutes at least once a week, Dr. Block suggests. The heat will penetrate the pelvis and increase blood flow, reducing muscle spasms and, possibly, swelling.

STRESS

Control Is the Cure

The kids are screaming, your car won't start, the big meeting is today, and it looks like you'll be late, plus you have a nasty cold. It's only 7:14 A.M., and you're just about ready to quit life. Aren't you a little young to be feeling so ragged all the time?

"Stress will do that to you," says Leah J. Dickstein, M.D., professor of psychiatry at the University of Louisville in Kentucky and former president of the American Medical Women's Association. "It can really wear you out. And the real problem is that you could be paving the way for other troubles later on."

The American Institute of Stress in Yonkers, New York, estimates that 90 percent of all visits to doctors are for stress-related disorders. Stress has been linked to a laundry list of diseases, including fatigue, hair loss, heart disease, high blood pressure, stroke, cancer, insomnia, low libido, lack of orgasm, and even impotence. "Stress speeds up your entire system and produces conditions in younger people that are more commonly associated with growing old," says Allen J. Elkin, Ph.D., director of the Stress Management and Counseling Center in New York City. "Virtually no part of your body can escape the ravages of stress."

Stress Busters

In today's world, you may feel that stress is almost inevitable, but there are ways to escape or reduce it. Here's how.

Work it out. Nothing eases stress more than exercise, according to David S. Holmes, Ph.D., professor of psychology at the University of Kansas in Lawrence. "Regular aerobic workouts reduce stress more effectively than meditation, psychiatric intervention, biofeedback, and conventional stress management," he says.

Exercise helps burn off all the stress-related chemicals in your system. During a workout, your body will also release mind-relaxing endorphins, Dr. Holmes says. And exercise strengthens your heart, too, further protecting you against the ravages of stress.

Don't be listless. So many projects, so little time. To beat stress, you have to learn to prioritize, according to Lee Reinert, Ph.D., director and lecturer for the Brandywine Biobehavioral Center, a counseling center in Downingtown, Pennsylvania. At the start of each day, pick the single most important task to complete, then finish it. If you're a person who makes to-do lists, never write one with more than five items. That way, you're more likely to get everything done, and you'll feel a greater sense of accomplishment and control, Dr. Reinert says. Then you can go ahead and make a second five-item list. While you're at it, make a list of things that you can delegate to co-workers and family members. "Remember: You don't have to do everything by yourself," Dr. Reinert says. "You can find help and support from people around you."

Just say no. Sometimes you have to learn to draw the line. "Stressed-out people often can't assert themselves," says Joan Lerner, Ph.D., a counseling psychologist at the University of Pennsylvania Counseling Service in Philadelphia. "And so they swallow things. Instead of saying, 'I don't want to do this' or 'I need some help,' they do it all themselves. Then they have even more to do."

Give your boss a choice. "Say, 'I'd really like to take this on, but I can't do that without giving up something else,'" says Merrill Douglass, a doctor of business administration and president of the Time Management Center in Marietta, Georgia, a company that trains individuals and corporations in the efficient use of time and energy, and co-author of *Manage Your Time, Manage Your Work, Manage Yourself.* "'Which of these things would you like me to do?'" Most bosses can take the hint, Dr. Douglass says. The same strategy works at home with your spouse, children, relatives, and friends.

Pad your schedule. "Realize that nearly everything will take longer than you anticipate," says Richard Swenson, M.D., author of *Margin: How to Create the Emotional, Physical, Financial, and Time Reserves You Need.* By allotting yourself enough time to accomplish a task, you cut back on anxiety. In general, if meeting deadlines is a problem, always give yourself 20 percent more time than you think you need to do the task.

Get a grip. Keep a hand exerciser or a tennis ball in your desk at work and give it a few squeezes during tense times. "When stress shoots adrenaline into the bloodstream, that calls for muscle action," says Roger Cady, M.D., medical director of the Shealy Institute for Comprehensive Health Care in Springfield, Missouri. "Squeezing something provides a release that satisfies our bodies' fight-or-flee response."

Practice your snorkeling. Want to really relax your muscles? Soak in a hot tub. To get the most relaxation from a hot bath, soak for 15 minutes in water that's just a few degrees warmer than your body temperature, or about 100° to 101°F.

When you're stressed out, carb up. If you want to unwind at the end of the day, eat a meal high in carbohydrates, says Judith Wurtman, Ph.D., a research scientist at the Massachusetts Institute of Technology and author of *Managing Your Mind and Mood through Food*. Carbohydrates trigger release of the brain neurotransmitter serotonin, which soothes you. Good sources of carbohydrates include rice, pasta, potatoes, breads, air-popped popcorn, and low-cal cookies.

Crack up. Humor is a proven stress reducer. Experts say a good laugh relaxes tense muscles, speeds more oxygen into your system, and lowers your blood pressure. So tune in to your favorite sitcom on television. Read a funny book. Call a friend and chuckle for a few minutes. It even helps to force a laugh once in a while. You'll find your stress melting away almost instantly.

Hold your breath. This technique should help you relax in 30 seconds. Take a deep breath and keep it in. Holding your hands palm to palm, press your fingers together. Wait 5 seconds, then slowly exhale through your lips while letting your hands relax. Do this five or six times until you unwind.

Take a 10-minute holiday. Meditation is a great stress reliever, but sometimes it's hard to find the time or place. Dr. Reinert suggests taking a mini-vacation right at your desk or kitchen table instead. Just close your eyes, breathe deeply (from your stomach), and picture yourself lying on a beach in Mexico. Feel the warmth of the sun. Hear the waves. Smell the salt air. "Just put a little distance between yourself and your stress," Dr. Reinert says. "A few minutes a day can be a great help."

Sound out stress. Try listening to gentle music, with flutes or other soft-sounding instruments, says Emmett Miller, M.D., a nationally known stress expert and medical director of the Cancer Support and Education Center in Menlo Park, California. He also suggests taking walks in quiet places and listening to leaves rustle or streams babble. Recordings of ocean waves or gentle rainstorms also help, he says.

Be a quitter. Look at your life. Are you doing too much? If you're on the company softball team, coaching Little League, volunteering on a church committee, and chauffeuring kids to piano lessons and Girl Scout outings and you don't have a weeknight free, you're choking on more than you can chew. "Prune your activity branches," suggests Dr. Swenson. Decide what gives you the most pleasure, and do only those things.

TELEVISION ADDICTION

Pandora's Electronic Box

Karen Dykeman's social life was crammed into a 19-inch box in her living room. She ate breakfast with Regis Philbin, lunch with Phil Donahue, dinner with Dan Rather, and a midnight snack with David Letterman.

"My life revolved around television virtually from first thing in the morning to late at night," says the 35-year-old switchboard operator in Seven Lakes, North Carolina. "Thank God, I've gotten away from that. Since I gave up watching television, I've lost 60 pounds, gotten involved in a community theater group, gone back to college, started dating, and just had a great time. I have a real life now. I definitely feel more vigorous and feel like I think more clearly."

Dykeman's energetic lifestyle since she kicked her TV habit comes as no shock to doctors who have long suspected that television's magnetic appeal saps us of our youth in many ways.

"There's absolutely no question that large amounts of TV viewing can make you feel old and weary before your time," says Kurt V. Gold, M.D., a physical medicine and rehabilitation physician at Immanuel Medical Center in Omaha, Nebraska, who has studied the effects of TV viewing on children. "Just think about what happens when you watch television. You're sitting passively, not using your muscles much . . . as a result, your muscles sag, and your mind stagnates. It's common sense. If you don't use it, you lose it."

But the danger of television isn't confined just to losing muscle tone or abusing brain cells. Some researchers also believe there is a definite link between heavy TV viewing and that dreaded middle-age bulge. A study of 800 adults, published in the *Journal of the American Dietetic Association*, found that the incidence of obesity among those watching an hour or less of television a day was 4.5 percent, but prevalence shot up to 19.2 percent among those watching four or more hours a day.

Excessive TV watching can also affect your cholesterol levels. In a study of 11,947 adults, Larry A. Tucker, Ph.D., professor and director of health promotion at Brigham Young University in Provo, Utah, found that people who watched three to four hours of television a day had twice the risk of developing high cholesterol levels as people who watched less than an hour a day. Excessive blood cholesterol is a risk factor for cardiovascular disease.

Turning It Off

Here are a few ways that you can control your television rather than having it control you.

Set boundaries. Put a limit on the amount of time you will watch each week and stick to it. "You need to set limits, or your viewing can easily get out of control," Dr. Tucker says.

Have an off-night. Make the television off-limits one night a week. See what creative things you and your family can find to do, Dr. Tucker says.

Be your own guide. Browse through a programming schedule and mark one or two programs an evening that you want to watch. Turn on the set when the show begins and turn it off immediately after it ends, Dr. Tucker says. This will discourage you from getting hooked on the next program.

Watch yourself. Before you turn on the television to watch a program, take a moment to visualize yourself walking over to the set and turning it off once the show is over. "That will program it into your brain that the television will actually go off at that time, and you will find something else to do," says Jane M. Healy, Ph.D., an educational psychologist in Vail, Colorado, and author of *Endangered Minds: Why Our Children Don't Think and What We Can Do about It.*

Reward yourself for not watching. For every hour that you don't watch television when you normally would, give yourself a point.

After you've accumulated 10 or 20 points, treat yourself with tickets to a play, an evening at a comedy club, or a dinner out with your family or friends, suggests Leonard Jason, Ph.D., professor of clinical and community psychology at DePaul University in Chicago.

Say what? Try turning on the set but turning off the sound, says Dr. Healy. More than likely, you'll quickly find something else to do with your time. "Much of the enticement of television comes from the sound track," says Dr. Healy.

Move it out of sight. Try putting your television in an unusual place, such as a cluttered room with no chairs, so you have to make an effort to watch it. "I've been remodeling my house, and I've put a bunch of furniture in front of my set, so I can't get to it very easily," Dr. Gold says. "You know what's nice? I've been working on my yard and spending time with my family instead of the television."

Get out of the house. Take a stroll or go to the pool for a leisurely swim. Get out into the real world. "If you watch three hours of television, do you usually feel invigorated? Probably not. If you go out for a 15-minute walk, you'll get a chance to talk to your neighbors and get some fresh air. I'll bet you'll come home feeling energized and ready to do anything but watch television," says C. Noel Bairey Merz, M.D., medical director of the Preventive and Rehabilitative Cardiac Center at Cedars-Sinai Medical Center in Los Angeles.

Call on me. "Arrange to have a friend phone you at the end of your favorite program. That might be all the incentive you need to break your habit, because once you get pulled away from the set, it's going to be easier not to go back to it," Dr. Healy says.

Get a hobby. "Find something that interests you, whether it be sketching, photography, caring for pets, or going to school," says Dykeman. "I got involved in things such as theater that made me feel important, needed, and useful. If you find something useful in your life, you can break the TV habit really quickly."

TYPE A
PERSONALITY

A Is for Attitude

You have never liked losing—not at the office, not on the tennis court, not even when your kid gets lucky and beats you at Monopoly. And you don't like wasting time either—especially when it's because of something you can't control, such as a slow-moving driver on the freeway or a slow-talking co-worker. With all the hurdles life puts in your path, it's no wonder you can't hold your temper anymore.

Whoa! Time out! These are some of the classic signs of Type A behavior. If you're running your motor at 150 miles per hour, 24 hours a day, it may be time to re-examine some goals and habits and your outlook on life. Because if you don't, you could be setting yourself up for problems—from headache to heart disease—that will erode your body's youthful edge.

"Type A behavior is very hard on your system," says C. David Jenkins, Ph.D., professor of preventive medicine and community health at the University of Texas Medical Branch at Galveston. "You're putting yourself under a lot of needless pressure. And believe me, that will take its toll in the long run, in ways you may not expect."

Type A people have six main characteristics. They love competition, attempt to achieve many poorly defined goals, have a strong need for recognition and advancement, are always in a hurry, show intense concentration and alertness, and are prone to anger.

In terms of aging, the key problem with Type A behavior is stress. Hard-driving people put themselves under constant pressure, and their bodies react by producing extra amounts of stress-related hormones. These hormones may cause long-term damage. A study of about 500 men and women at Harvard Medical School showed that Type A's had a 50 percent higher risk of suffering heart attacks than the less intense Type B's.

Mellowing Out

You can't really "cure" Type A personality, Dr. Jenkins says. Not that you'd want to; there's really nothing wrong with a touch of assertiveness and a sturdy work ethic. But you may want to change some daily habits and attitudes to help lower your risk of Type A health trouble. Here are a few suggestions to get started.

Aim lower. Sure, you want to succeed at everything. But there are only 24 hours in a day—and sometimes something has to give. So be a little more choosy. "I think setting realistic goals is the most important thing a Type A person can do," says Lee Reinert, Ph.D., director and lecturer for the Brandywine Biobehavioral Center, a counseling center in Downingtown, Pennsylvania. At the start of each week, make a list of things you feel you absolutely must do. Each time you write something down, ask yourself what would happen if you didn't do it. If you can't come up with a legitimate concern, scratch that item off the list. Now comes the tough part: Cut the final list by five items. You may try delegating a few of the items to your spouse, children, or co-workers. "What's left is a more achievable set of tasks," Dr. Reinert says. "You'll get a greater sense of accomplishment this way, and you won't be chasing after brushfires that keep popping up."

Try aerobics. You'll sweat the stress a little less if you work out regularly. Aerobic exercise relieves stress and can ward off its long-term consequences, says David S. Holmes, Ph.D., professor of psychology at the University of Kansas in Lawrence.

One word of caution, however: Don't overdo it. Because they tend to overtrain, Type A people are injured more during exercise, reports *Sports Medicine Digest.* "Get a good workout. Raise your heart rate, but don't try to win at all costs. Don't keep trying to beat your own record," Dr. Jenkins says.

Account for your anger. Keeping journals helps people discover the roots of their aggressiveness and anger, Dr. Reinert says. "A lot of times, you're not really mad at what's going on right now. You're upset about more of a core issue—maybe an unhappy family relationship," she says. Writing down your thoughts and feelings may help you discover what's really angering you. It can also help you detect patterns. Maybe you always get mad when you're waiting in line. Or when Marla in accounting won't let you get a word in at the staff meeting. If you anticipate these moments, you can either find ways to avoid them or ask yourself whether they're really important enough to blow your stack over.

Make amends. Is that little old lady in the slow-moving Buick really trying to make you mad? Was she awake deep into the night plotting ways to make you late? Or is she just a little old lady who needs to use some extra caution to drive these days? Redford B. Williams, M.D., professor of psychiatry and director of the Behavioral Research Center at Duke University Medical Center in Durham, North Carolina, suggests putting yourself in the other person's shoes. When you look at the world from the perspective of the people who anger you, you'll probably be a little less cynical about them—and a little less Type A in the process. Dr. Williams also suggests doing some volunteer work as a way to relieve hostility and gain empathy for other people.

Come up for air. Type A people typically schedule their days to the millisecond. That leaves no margin for error—and sets them up for extra stress when things go wrong. So try to give yourself a 10 percent pad. If you work a 10-hour day, leave at least an hour free to deal with the unexpected. If that sounds like an awfully big block of time, Dr. Reinert suggests setting aside five or six minutes per hour instead. These cooldown periods can help you organize your thoughts and create new plans of attack. They can also spark creativity, making the rest of the workday more productive, she says.

Pay attention to your body. Find another 10 or 15 minutes a day to check in with your body. Sit on a comfortable chair in a quiet room, close your eyes, and breathe deeply. Tense, then release, the muscles in your feet. Then do your calves. Work up your body, paying special attention to the areas that feel tight or are throbbing (especially your shoulders and neck). "This is a great stress reducer," Dr. Reinert says. "It lets your body relax. And it shows you how needlessly tense you become during the day."

VARICOSE VEINS

You Don't Have to Live with Them

Who doesn't hate varicose veins, whether they're small and spidery or bulgy blue ropes? Varicose veins creep up the legs of over half of us after age 40, and they're a potent reminder of aging. For women, wearing shorts or a swimsuit becomes a problem. Men have it a little better cosmetically, since hair and pants legs pretty much cover them up.

Medically, though, they can be a source of discomfort and pain to anyone who has them. They can throb and feel heavy, making you feel like you're dragging your legs around. They can cause chronic aching in the calves. At night, they can cause legs to cramp or feel restless, disturbing your much-needed sleep. They can even itch and feel sore. And although it's rare, varicose veins can indicate a clot in a deeper leg vein.

Heredity and female hormones during pregnancy play a role in causing varicose veins, as do lifestyle factors like a low-fiber diet and smoking. Also, many people with varicose veins have an inherited weakness in the valves inside the leg veins. These valves normally prevent blood from leaking back down as it flows up to the heart. If a valve leaks, gravity forces blood into lower veins when you stand up. Once this process is repeated enough times, the vein walls can become permanently stretched.

Preventive Measures

If varicose veins run in the family but haven't yet turned up on you, there are several things you can do to help forestall them.

Pare off some pounds. If you're significantly overweight, a gradual, healthy weight-loss plan can be your veins' biggest ally, says Alan Kanter, M.D., medical director of the Vein Center of Orange County in Irvine, California. Extra pounds put unnecessary pressure on your legs.

Fiber up your diet. Make sure your diet is high in fiber to keep your bowels healthy and stools soft. This will prevent straining due to constipation, Dr. Kanter says, and this straining can often increase vein pressure and cause varicose veins. Fiber is found in abundance in fruits, vegetables, and whole grains.

Drink water. Another way to soften stools is to be sure you're well-hydrated by drinking at least eight glasses of water a day, says Dr. Kanter.

Don't smoke. Or if you do, stop, says Glenn Geelhoed, M.D., professor of surgery and international medical education at George Washington University Medical Center in Washington, D.C. Smoking increases your risk of developing underlying vein disease, which can contribute to varicose veins, he says.

Lift weights wisely. Weight-lifting exercise will help with weight control, but you need to do it right to avoid encouraging a vein problem, says Dr. Kanter. Use smaller weights and do more repetitions rather than straining with heavy weights, he says. Ask a trainer to set up a program for you.

Jog on gentle ground. Plan your running route along soft surfaces such as dirt, grass, or a cinder track whenever possible, Dr. Kanter suggests. The impact of running on pavement can aggravate vein swelling.

Keep moving on the job. Don't sit for two or three hours straight while you work, says Malcolm O. Perry, M.D., professor and chief of vascular surgery at Texas Tech University Health Sciences Center in Lubbock. Be sure to get up and move around often to keep blood circulating.

Home Treatment for the Ones You Have

If you already have a few varicose veins developing, here's how to keep them under control.

Sleep on a slope. Put six- by six-inch blocks under the foot of your bed and leave them there, says Dr. Perry. This keeps blood from pooling in your legs at night. You can quickly adapt to the tilt.

Wear support hose. For a few small veins, choose high-quality support hose from a good clothing store or drugstore and wear them regularly, says Dr. Perry. These are available for both men and women. For men, support hose are available in knee-high lengths. For women, they are available in knee-high, stocking, and panty-hose styles. The slight compression will help keep the veins down, he says.

Try gradient stockings. If the veins you have are fairly large, even good-quality support hose aren't enough, says Dr. Perry. Ask your doctor to prescribe custom-fitted gradient compression stockings instead. "They're hot and heavy, but they help," he says. Most women opt to wear them under pants for work and save the more sheer support hose for special occasions.

The Big Cover-Up

There are two basic medical treatments available for varicose veins: sclerotherapy (injection) and surgical removal (stripping).

Sclerotherapy involves injecting a solution into a vein that causes the vein's walls to be absorbed by the body. No anesthesia is needed, and "you can be up and about your business right afterward," says David Green, M.D., a dermatologist at the Varicose Vein Center in Bethesda, Maryland. A few weeks to months later, the vein shrivels to an invisible thread of scar tissue under the skin.

The cost usually ranges from around $100 to several hundred dollars, depending on the number of injections needed. Multiple treatments may be required if you have many affected veins.

Surgical stripping is another procedure that is sometimes recommended for severe varicose veins. Many patients have the surgery as outpatients, going home late the same day. Even though the affected veins are completely removed, there is no risk to your circulation because other vessels can easily compensate for the loss of the superficial veins, Dr. Perry says.

While some scarring usually results from surgery, often long lengths of vein can be removed through several tiny incisions.

What are the advantages of surgery? Many vein specialists say that even large varicose veins can be effectively treated with sclerotherapy. But some vascular surgeons point out that there is a high rate of recurrence with the injection treatment, and multiple visits are often required if you have many affected veins. However, when ultrasound imaging is used to help guide the surgery, preliminary results show a higher success rate in fewer visits.

VISION CHANGES

Set Your Sights High

You've booked the corner table at Chez Chic, and it's time to wow the clients from out of town. The sommelier hands you the wine list. You sigh nonchalantly and open the list with a practiced touch of disdain.

Uh-oh. You can't read it. Your eyes won't focus on the fine print. So much for being nonchalant. You straighten your arms, hold the list a yard from your face and start to squint.

Just like that, you've gone from high-powered deal maker to dear old grandma or grandpa, sitting there reading a large-print version of *The Old Farmer's Almanac*. What's next—trifocals and a rocking chair?

It's a fact of life that sooner or later, your vision is going to fade a bit. Nine out of 10 people between ages 40 and 64 wear glasses or contact lenses to make reading and other close work a little easier. But don't despair. You may be able to slow the process with regular eye exams and a healthy diet, and you can also take steps now to deal with serious vision problems such as glaucoma, cataracts, and macular degeneration that could lead to greatly reduced sight or even blindness.

Up Close and Blurry

One of the most common age-related eye problems is a form of farsightedness called presbyopia, and it's as inevitable as rain at a picnic. "There's really no way around it," says Richard Bensinger, M.D., an ophthalmologist in Seattle and spokesman for the American Academy of Ophthalmology. "It's easy to correct, but it means you're probably going to have to wear glasses or contact lenses."

In addition to presbyopia, spots and floaters may appear more often as you get older. These are little specks or dots that pop up occasionally in your field of vision, then disappear after an hour or a day or more. "Usually, it's nothing serious," Dr. Bensinger says. "The spots just drift down out of your vision, and that's it. But if you suddenly see lots of spots or flashes of light in your eyes, that could be a sign that something more serious is wrong, and you should see a doctor immediately."

Taking the Long View

Barring accidental injury, your eyes will probably serve you well right up to your midsixties. You may need a new set of reading glasses every few years, but you probably won't notice any serious deterioration of vision.

Still, experts warn that you should never take your eyes for granted. Most serious eye diseases are painless and show no symptoms for years. If you don't have your eyes examined on a regular basis, you may not know how bad things have gotten until it's too late to help. Here are some diseases to watch out for.

GLAUCOMA. This progressive disease causes 12 percent of all blindness in America. It is marked by increased fluid pressure in the eye that, over the years, can cause irreversible damage to the nerves that send vision impulses to your brain.

Doctors don't know what causes most kinds of glaucoma, and they don't know how to cure it. Vision lost to glaucoma cannot be restored, but when detected early enough, glaucoma can be controlled through eyedrops, oral tablets, laser surgery, or even an artificial drain created by eye surgeons, all of which allow the fluid to escape and lower pressure.

An estimated 3 million Americans have glaucoma, and half of them don't even know it. Another 5 to 10 million people have the pressure buildup that precedes the disease, and far fewer than half of them know it. The best advice for dealing with glaucoma? Find out if you have it—now. "The earlier this disease is picked up, the better able we'll—to control it," says Carl Kupfer, M.D., director of the National Eye Institute in Bethesda, Maryland. That means regular eye exams, especially if you're at high risk for glaucoma.

CATARACTS. Although they usually don't become a problem until you near retirement age, cataracts often start forming much earlier in life, especially if you have ever had an eye injury or have undergone radiation treatments, chemotherapy, or an organ transplant.

Over the years, the once-clear lens in each eye may turn yellow because of protein buildup. In time, the lens may become milky white and translucent, clouding vision to the point where you need an artificial lens implant. This plastic replacement lens does not flex to focus light as the original lens did, but with corrective glasses, your vision can be restored quite well. "While we can't yet cure cataracts, we can certainly provide patients with good sight," Dr. Bensinger says.

Cataracts, like glaucoma, may have a hereditary link. So if anyone in your family has had cataracts, you may be at higher risk and should have your eyes examined more often than the standard every three years.

MACULAR DEGENERATION. This insidious eye disease robs you of your fine visual skills. "In more advanced cases, you would be able to tell that someone was standing in front of you, but you couldn't tell who it was," Dr. Bensinger says. "You could see that there was a bus coming down the street, but you couldn't tell which one because you couldn't read the sign."

Unfortunately, there's little hope right now for restoring sight lost to macular degeneration, although laser surgery may help stabilize sight for a time. There is some hopeful news, though: Because macular degeneration strikes people over age 60 almost exclusively, you can start now—perhaps with the help of an improved diet—to ward it off before it starts.

DIABETIC RETINOPATHY. As its name implies, retinopathy primarily strikes people with diabetes. It is the leading cause of blindness in people ages 20 to 50. Loss of vision begins to occur when blood vessels in the back of the eye leak, blurring vision and sometimes denying nutrients to the eye.

"If you have diabetes," Dr. Bensinger says, "I cannot urge you strongly enough to have your eyes checked regularly. It can literally save your sight."

"Early detection of diabetic retinopathy is even more of a success story than testing for glaucoma," Dr. Kupfer says. If it's caught early, there's a 95 percent chance that you can keep your sight for at least five years, he says.

Focusing on Prevention

You can't change your genes, so there's not much you can do about the biggest vision risk factor of all—heredity. Still, here's some advice to give you the best chance of staying 20/20 into the twenty-first century.

Get your eyes checked. Doctors just can't say this enough. "Regular eye examinations are by far the most important thing you can do to help preserve your vision," Dr. Bensinger says.

If you are between ages 30 and 50 and have no previous eye problems, the American Academy of Ophthalmology suggests seeing an ophthalmologist every three years. If you have a family history of glaucoma or diabetes or are already wearing glasses or contact lenses, your doctor may suggest more frequent visits.

The academy suggests an immediate visit to the doctor if you have any of the following symptoms: sudden vision changes in one or both eyes, unexplainable redness, seeing a number of spots or floaters or showers of sparks in the corners of your eyes, eye pain that won't go away, or accidental contact with chemicals, especially lye.

Hide behind some shades. Sunglasses that block both UVA and UVB rays and visible blue light may help decrease the risk of cataracts, Dr. Bensinger says. Wraparound glasses that cover the sides of your eyes are a good idea since they shield your eyes completely. And try to wear a hat with a visor to block direct sunlight from your eyes.

"Exposure to sunlight drops the age at which you may develop cataracts," Dr. Bensinger says. "So if you're going to be outside, it makes sense to cut that sunlight as much as possible."

Stop smoking. Cancer. Wrinkles. Stinky clothes. Yellow teeth. Emphysema. If you really need another reason to quit, here it is: Cigarette smoking might cause cataracts. A Harvard Medical School study of 120,000 nurses showed that women who smoke 35 or more cigarettes a day have a 63 percent greater risk of developing cataracts. While the reason isn't known, researchers speculate that smoking may reduce antioxidant levels in your blood, promoting cataract growth.

Try some see-food. The links between diet and vision are still weak. But antioxidants—vitamins C and E plus beta-carotene—showed promise as cataract fighters in the Harvard Nurses' Health Study. A report in the *American Journal of Clinical Nutrition* claimed that people who eat 3½ servings of fruits and vegetables every day have a lower risk of cataracts, too.

"Eating a healthy diet may delay the usual aging of the lens and so delay cataracts," says Paul F. Jacques, Sc.D., epidemiologist with the Jean Mayer USDA Human Nutrition Research Center on Aging at Tufts University in Boston.

WRINKLES

Draw the Line on Early Lines

You pop out of bed for a healthy, fat-free breakfast, followed by five quick miles on your exercise bike. Then you hit the shower, feeling like you just had a drink from the fountain of youth. You finish, wrap a towel around yourself, and peek at your million-dollar face in the mirror. Hold it. Where did all those wrinkles come from? Around the eyes, the smile lines—all of a sudden, you feel like you're turning into your mom or dad.

You feel old. And maybe less attractive. Well, before you give up the workouts and trade the bike in for a rocking chair, know this—with today's technology, you actually can look on the outside like the gorgeous young thing you are on the inside. Between some treatments that you can do at home and your doctor's help, you can repair or erase most of your wrinkles. And you can easily prevent new wrinkles from forming.

Do-It-Yourself Wrinkle Removal

Here's how to rid yourself of wrinkles on your own.

Look for alpha hydroxy acids (AHAs). These naturally occurring acids—derived from plants, fruits, and other food products, such as sugarcane (glycolic acid) and sour milk (lactic acid)—can be found in over-the-counter creams, lotions, and gels. They improve sun-damaged skin by exfoliating dead skin cells on the skin's surface and uncovering the younger cells underneath. They also plump up the skin, in essence filling in the "dents" we know as wrinkles. Glycolic acid is the most widely used AHA.

Use an 8 percent AHA preparation on your face and neck twice a day—once in the morning and once at night, says Lorrie J. Klein, M.D., a dermatologist in private practice in Laguna Niguel, California. For the sensitive area around the eyes, use a fragrance-free 5 percent AHA eye cream.

Consider beta hydroxy acid. Some people with sensitive skin find AHAs too irritating. If that's the case, try using salicylic acid, known as beta hydroxy acid, instead. Available in moisturizers and cleansers such as Oil of Olay's Age-Defying Series, beta hydroxy acid exfoliates the skin and reduces the signs of lines and wrinkles just as AHAs do but with less irritation, says Debra Price, M.D., clinical assistant professor of dermatology at the University of Miami School of Medicine.

"C" your way to smoother skin. Unlike alpha hydroxy and beta hydroxy acid products, which reverse skin damage by speeding up the exfoliation process, vitamin C might help prevent damage in the first place. As an antioxidant, vitamin C fights off free radicals, unstable molecules that form when the skin is exposed to sunlight and ultraviolet radiation. (Free radicals "steal" electrons from the body's healthy molecules, harming cells and leading to premature wrinkling and other forms of damage.) Vitamin C also helps the body produce new collagen, a protein that keeps skin smooth and firm. Unfortunately, the sun robs the skin of vitamin C right when it needs it most, according to Lorraine Meisner, Ph.D., professor of preventive medicine at the University of Wisconsin Medical School in Madison.

Because of this, you should apply topical vitamin C daily—with a sunscreen—before significant sun exposure. One topical vitamin C product is Cellex-C, a 10 percent vitamin C solution available without a prescription from dermatologists and licensed aestheticians. Cellex-C also contains zinc (a trace mineral) and tyrosine (an amino acid), which help the vitamin penetrate the skin's surface, according to Dr. Meisner, who is co-inventor of the patented formulation in Cellex-C. The solution provides your skin with 20 times the amount of vitamin C that you would get from your diet.

The ABCs of Wrinkle Repair

The natural route isn't the only way to go to get rid of wrinkles. Dermatologists have developed a brand-new bag of tricks to make wrinkles disappear, ranging from prescription creams and peelings to surface repairs and surgery. Here are some medical options.

Smooth them with Retin-A. Tretinoin (Retin-A), an acne medication derived from vitamin A, has earned its reputation as an excellent wrinkle smoother, particularly for the fine lines caused by years of indulging in the sun. It's available only through a prescription, and there are three types of Retin-A prescribed by doctors: regular Retin-A, Retin-A Micro, and Renova. The kind you use depends on your skin type, so consult your dermatologist before choosing. Using it is very simple: Apply a pea-size amount to your face and the backs of your hands every night. Tretinoin penetrates the damaged skin cells and spurs them to start making collagen again, which fills in fine wrinkles.

"It doesn't erase severe damage, but it does erase fine lines," says Edward Jeffes, M.D., associate professor of dermatology at the University of California, Irvine. But be patient: It takes at least six months to see the full benefits.

Zap 'em. More doctors are using lasers—concentrated light that can cut tissue and destroy some tumors—to smooth wrinkles. The laser emits a rapid series of beams that are half the size of a pencil eraser. The wrinkle is vaporized during a series of sharply directed, split-second exposures. Lasers work best on wrinkles on the lower and upper lips, the eyelids, and the backs of the hands, says Laurence David, M.D., president of the International Society of Cosmetic Laser Surgeons in Hermosa Beach, California.

Peel away the lines. Chemical peels are another procedure for smoothing out wrinkles. A dermatologist applies a chemical such as glycolic acid, lactic aid, trichloroacetic acid, salicylic acid, or phenol, alone or in combination, and your skin reacts to this by sloughing off several layers of skin cells. Then new skin is regenerated that not only looks better but is also less prone to skin cancer. The strength and type of solution that the doctor uses determines whether it's a light peel, which affects light surface wrinkles, or a deep peel, which works on the deeper wrinkles. The deeper the peel, the more intricate the procedure. Just remember that after peels, your skin is a lot more vulnerable to sunlight, so sunscreen is a necessity.

Fill 'em up. Plumping up the skin beneath a wrinkle is an alternative to peeling off wrinkles from the surface, says Gary Monheit, M.D., assistant professor of dermatology at the University of Alabama School of Medicine in Birmingham. Dermatologists use several substances as wrinkle fillers, but the best-known is cattle-derived collagen. Collagen is a fibrous tissue that forms a supporting network just under the surface of the skin. The doctor injects the collagen into your wrinkle, and a lump appears above the skin surface. When the lump fades (in as little as six hours), the wrinkle will have been smoothed away.

The problems with collagen? It's temporary—results last from 4 to 15 months, Dr. Monheit says. And some people may be allergic to this form of collagen, so the doctor must first perform an allergy test.

Stopping Them before They Start

The two main causes of wrinkles are sun damage and smoking, and unless you move to another galaxy, you're not going to completely avoid either one. Here's how you can keep both of them from leaving their mark on you.

Put up a chemical parasol. Sunscreen is your number one weapon against sun damage, says Albert M. Kligman, M.D., professor of dermatology at the University of Pennsylvania School of Medicine in Philadelphia. Use a full-spectrum sunscreen that blocks both kinds of ultraviolet radiation (UVA and UVB), and use it every day, year-round, Dr. Kligman says. After you cleanse your skin in the morning, leave it slightly damp and apply pea-size dabs of sunscreen on your cheeks and forehead, working it into the skin all over your face. Don't forget the backs of your hands, neck, and décolletage. If you use Retin-A or another type of topical anti-wrinkle cream, sunscreen is essential because these creams make your skin more sensitive to sunlight. Put it on after you've applied the cream. Be sure to use a sunscreen with a sun protection factor (SPF) of 15 or higher.

Dump that nasty habit. Sorry, no high-tech solution or miracle herb can help you here. Smoking is a prime line maker, and the only way to prevent getting wrinkles from tobacco smoke is by quitting and avoiding secondhand smoke.

No aerobics for your face. Although facial exercises have been touted in many beauty books, most of them actually increase wrinkling, says Karen Burke, M.D., Ph.D., a dermatologist in private practice in New York City. When you grimace or contort your face through exercises, you are working the same muscles that caused wrinkles in the first place, she says.

Sleep on your back. "It's the best position for a younger-looking, unlined face," says Dr. Monheit. If you've been burrowing into your pillow face-first for years, lying on your back every night with a pillow under your knees may help you to change the habit, he says.

Part II
The Age Rejuvenators

ADVENTURE

Reach for Your Outer Limits

For her vacation one summer, Anne Bancroft went to Antarctica, where a balmy day is about −23°F. Then she and three other women spent 67 days pulling 200-pound sleds for 660 miles into headwinds up to 50 miles per hour to reach the South Pole. Why?

"A trip like this rejuvenates you," says Bancroft, a 38-year-old motivational speaker and polar explorer from St. Paul, Minnesota, who was the first woman to trek across the ice to both poles. "You're in the best shape of your life, and there's something wonderful about that. You get the feeling when you get back home and into the craziness of life that you're going to live a lot longer because you did have an adventure like that. It makes you feel strong and good."

Now, of course, you don't have to cross miles of barren ice to feel younger, but doctors do say that if you're truly looking for a fountain of youth, you should try tossing more adventure into your life.

"Adventure and risk-taking can make you feel and think like a person who is years younger. It's believed that when you have thrill-seeking adventures, there's a release of certain chemicals in the brain that are truly uplifting to mood," says psychiatrist Bernard Vittone, M.D., director of the National Center for the Treatment of Phobias, Anxiety, and Depression in Washington, D.C.

But other experts suspect that adventure does more than just jump-start your emotions.

"Any time you are re-energized in a vibrant way, as through an adventure, there are very positive physiological effects, including increased blood and oxygen flow to the tissues in your body. That, along with the emotional effects of rediscovering your life's energy, can make some people literally look younger," says Mark Weaver, Ph.D., a psychologist with the Experiential Learning Institute in Oklahoma City.

"The importance of adventure isn't so much that you climbed a mountain, rafted on an unfamiliar river, or even started your own small business. The key point is to achieve something new and to discover how you can reach beyond your comfort zone and stretch yourself as a human being," Dr. Weaver says.

So why do some people feel the urge to explore the Amazon rain forest while others spend their evenings reading the fine print on their insurance policies? Some adventurousness is learned from your parents. "If you have parents who are always amplifying the danger of a situation, you'll learn to view situations as more threatening," Dr. Vittone says. "On the other hand, if you have parents who encourage adventure, you're going to develop a higher threshold of excitement."

But biology plays a role, too. "We all react differently to different types of stimulation," Dr. Vittone says. "There are certain anxiety centers in the brain that are tripped off more easily in some people than in others. So we all have our own threshold of adventure or risk-taking behavior that we feel comfortable doing."

As we age, these anxiety centers become more sensitive, and we gradually lose our ability to distinguish between the negative sort of anxiety that is associated with stress or tension and the more positive types of anxiety that are a natural and exciting part of experiencing something new, Dr. Vittone says. As a result, we become more fearful and begin avoiding any situations that produce anxiety, including relatively safe recreational adventures such as hiking.

"The problem is that people start viewing all those feelings of anxiety in the same negative way, instead of realizing that some anxiety can be positive," Dr. Vittone says. "It's that lumping of those positive and negative feelings together that makes people gravitate toward wanting to feel safe and comfortable all the time."

A Prescription for Thrills

That overwhelming desire for safety and comfort causes many of us to develop what some experts call stagnant spirits. Fortunately, you don't have to climb Mount Everest, become a mud wrestler, or take up hang gliding to get adventure into your life.

"Since we're all different, there's going to be a range of adventures that people find thrilling," Dr. Vittone says. "For some people, just driving to a new town and exploring may do it. For others, it may take parachuting. Whatever you do, it's that feeling of a thrill that you're looking for." Here are some ways to get more thrills into your day.

Let your mind wander. "Every adventure starts with curiosity," says Andrea Shrednick, Ph.D., a clinical psychologist in private practice in Los Angeles. "Allow your mind to wander free. Imagine if you had a week all to yourself. Where would you go? What would you do? What types of foods would you eat? If you allow yourself to daydream like that, it will whet your appetite for the real thing."

Know your limits. Take an honest look at your skills and abilities and see if they realistically match up with the adventure you have in mind. "A person who doesn't take a careful inventory of his skills and capabilities is a fool. That's being reckless, and recklessness is not virtuous," says Jasper S. Hunt Jr., Ph.D., director of adventure education programs in the department of educational leadership at Mankato State University in Minnesota and a leader of wilderness-survival outings for Outward Bound, an adventure-travel club.

Be prepared. "Every adventure, no matter how small, is a step-by-step process," Bancroft says. "We always know what we're facing before we get started on an expedition. You can't control Mother Nature, but before you start, you can test your gear, get yourself in shape, and do all the other things that make your chances of a successful trip far greater."

Take small steps. Start with simple adventures, then gradually increase the difficulty as your competence and confidence grow. If you want to learn to climb, for example, join a hiking club and build up your expertise before deciding to tackle Mount McKinley, Dr. Hunt says.

Accept reality. Don't push yourself into a dangerous situation. "If you look at mountaineers, for example, the ones who are still alive to tell about their adventures don't try to conquer the mountain at all costs. They do their homework and know when it's unsafe and time to back off. That's a good lesson for all of us to learn," Bancroft says.

Share your dreams. "If you're facing a scary challenge, tell someone about it," Bancroft advises. "I don't think any of us are very successful strictly by ourselves. We all need pats on the back and encouragement from others to fulfill our dreams."

Have some laughs. "For me, the best tool for getting through hard struggles is not taking myself too seriously," Bancroft says. "I don't think I could do any of this without a sense of humor. You tend to lose sight of the purpose of the adventure if you don't have fun."

AEROBIC EXERCISE

Move into the Future Youthfully

Aerobics classes have been one of the most popular activities at health clubs for quite a while—so much so that *aerobics* has become a buzzword for fitness. And that's fitting. Aerobics classes, which usually last from 20 minutes to an hour, rev up your heart and work your major muscle groups, improving your cardiovascular system and helping you become fit.

Besides structured classes, a whole range of exercises—biking, running, walking, and swimming, for example—also give you the aerobic edge. And they can do more than make you feel fit. They can make you feel younger, both today and in the years to come. In fact, when it comes to age erasers, aerobic exercise is right at the head of the list. Its benefits are wide-ranging.

Aerobic exercise helps combat aging by preventing heart disease, maintaining bone and muscle strength, and keeping your mind sharp. It may also play a role in fending off diabetes and certain forms of cancer. And it can help take the edge off daily stress by boosting your mood and energy level. Premenstrual syndrome (PMS) and menopausal symptoms are often reduced with exercise as well.

The effect of aerobic exercise on your heart and cardiovascular system is a major benefit. Cardiovascular disease is the number one killer of both men and women in the United States, and aerobic exercise helps decrease your risk, says Alan Mikesky, Ph.D., an exercise physiologist at Indiana University School of Physical Education in Indianapolis. That's the main reason that you should make exercise a priority, he says.

Aerobic exercise strengthens the heart and makes it more efficient. And at heart-pumping levels, exercise burns enough calories to reduce body fat, leading to weight loss. Keeping trim not only helps you feel better but also helps keep your blood pressure down, thus reducing another major risk factor for heart disease.

Further, exercise may help keep your cholesterol under control. Studies show that exercise increases high-density lipoprotein (HDL) cholesterol, the good type that helps sweep low-density lipoprotein (LDL) cholesterol, the bad type, from the arteries. High-intensity exercise has been shown to increase HDL levels by 5 to 15 percent.

Aerobic exercise is effective in preserving your bones as well. Weight-bearing exercise such as walking or running places stress on the bones, helping to maintain or increase bone strength. This is particularly important for postmenopausal women, who experience bone loss at the rate of 2 to 4 percent per year. Riding a bicycle, either stationary or moving, can also be effective.

The Immediate Return

Aerobic exercise can make you feel younger today by boosting your self-esteem and improving your mental attitude. Regular exercise produces several rewards—muscle strength, gains in your aerobic fitness level, feelings of control over your environment, and positive feedback from friends you exercise with—that can make you feel better about yourself.

Aerobic exercise can also help fight fatigue. "Despite what people sometimes feel, an exercise program tends to increase energy levels rather than decrease them," says William Simpson, M.D., professor of family medicine in the department of family medicine at the Medical University of South Carolina in Charleston. If you stop and pay attention to how you feel after exercise, you will recognize that you feel more alert and more energetic, and those feelings can carry over for several hours after the exercise session, he says.

With all of these benefits, it should come as no surprise that aerobic exercise may help you live longer. In a study of 3,120 adult women conducted by the Cooper Institute for Aerobics Research in Dallas, the higher the women's levels of physical fitness, the lower their death rates. And a follow-up to a Harvard study found that by the time they were 80 years old, men who had gotten adequate exercise between the ages of 35 and 79 lived one to two years longer than men who didn't get regular exercise.

Getting Started

The general guidelines for aerobic exercise have been to get 30 minutes of continuous aerobic exercise that gets your heart rate up to between 50 percent and 90 percent of your maximum at least three times a week. How high you need to raise your heart rate to reap anti-aging benefits depends on your age, sex, and current fitness level.

If getting that much exercise in whole blocks is difficult, try instead to log 30 minutes over the course of the day—by walking 10 minutes before work, 10 minutes at lunch, and 10 minutes after you get home, for example. There is growing evidence that it is the cumulative amount of activity, not the amount done at any one time, that can offer long-term health benefits.

It's one thing to know that you should exercise, but it's another to get going and stick with it. Here are some tips to help you out.

Get physical. A physical checkup, that is. If you're just starting an exercise program, see your doctor. During the examination, your doctor will assess your blood pressure and check to see if you have had any previous injuries to your muscles or bones that could be exacerbated by exercise. If you haven't exercised in the past, are over 35, and have risk factors for heart disease, your doctor may recommend a stress electrocardiogram or a treadmill test.

Get some guidance. When you first start your exercise program, it's very important to get supervision from someone who knows about exercise, says Janet P. Wallace, Ph.D., associate professor of kinesiology at Indiana University at Bloomington. On your own, you may tend to overdo it, so find a trainer to show you the right pace. Ask candidates if they have certification from the American College of Sports Medicine, the American Council on Exercise, the Aerobics and Fitness Association of America, or the National Strength and Conditioning Association.

Make it a priority. Instead of looking at exercise as a leisure activity, look at it as a necessity, says Dr. Mikesky. In other words, make an exercise appointment with yourself that can't be canceled, postponed, or rescheduled. Respect that appointment just as you would any other. This is another advantage to having a trainer, as your workouts will be scheduled.

Warm up. It's important to warm up and stretch before plunging headlong into your workout session. Warming up increases circulation to your muscles, makes them more pliable, and helps prevent injury, says physical therapist Mark Taranta, director of the Physical Therapy Practice in Philadelphia. Try walking, jogging slowly, or riding an exercise bike at a slow pace for a few minutes until you get a light sweat going. Then stretch for 8 to 10 minutes.

Make it fun. People are more successful at getting into a regular exercise program when they choose an activity they enjoy, says Dr. Wallace. If it's boring or too hard, you won't stick with it, so try different things until you find a type of exercise that you really like.

Mix it up. "Aerobic activities are not the most exciting activities," says Dr. Wallace, so try combining them with another activity that you like. If you enjoy racquetball or tennis (anaerobic activities), try walking for 15 minutes before or after. Or combine different types of aerobic activities. "If you're at the health club with a lot of aerobic equipment, move from one to the next," she says. Spending 10 minutes on each one will be less boring. So try the stair climber, the bike, and then the treadmill.

Couple up. Consider going to the gym with your partner, says Dr. Wallace. A study of 16 married couples at her institution found that the dropout rate for individuals who went to the gym with their spouses was much lower (6 percent) compared with those who went to the gym on their own (42 percent). You don't necessarily have to work out together; just go there together, she says.

Get in a group. If you really have trouble exercising on your own, aim for a group activity. Join an aerobics class or a running group. Start your own walking club with friends from work. Exercising with others will help you stick with it, says Joanne Stevenson, R.N., Ph.D., professor of nursing at Ohio State University College of Nursing in Columbus, because you'll have to answer for yourself. If you miss a class, someone will ask where you were, she says.

Give yourself a break. Getting into a regular exercise routine can take some time, so allow yourself to slip up here and there. Take it a week at a time, says Dr. Wallace. "If you blow it one day or one week, you still have next week," she says.

AFFIRMATIONS

Phrases That Sing Your Praises

Some days, everyone's a critic. Is it too much to ask for a little compliment once in a while? Well, instead of waiting for someone else, why not say something nice to yourself, an affirmation? They're short, positive phrases about you, your life, and your world. And experts say that repeating them daily can build self-esteem, give you a booster shot of vitality, and help you see things in a more optimistic light.

"There's so much negativity around that it tends to pull you down after a while," says Susan Jeffers, Ph.D., a psychologist in private practice in Tesuque, New Mexico, and author of *Feel the Fear and Do It Anyway*. "Affirmations can help you live a happier life and diminish the negative clutter that clouds your sense of purpose. They're extraordinarily powerful little pick-me-ups."

Affirmations also are surefire stress busters. "You should have a list of affirmations ready that you can start repeating when you feel stressed," says Emmett Miller, M.D., a nationally known stress expert and medical director of the Cancer Support and Education Center in Menlo Park, California. "They don't have to be complicated. Just thinking to yourself, 'I can handle this' or 'I know more about this than anyone here' will work. It pulls you away from the animal reflex to stress—the quick breathing, the cold hands—and toward the reasoned response—the intellect, the part of you that can really handle it."

The Power of Positive Talk

Before you start using affirmations, you must have two things. The first is patience. "It may take a while to overcome all the negativity you've built up," Dr. Jeffers says. "Some of the effects of affirmations are immediate—you'll start feeling a little more optimistic right away. But only with repetition can you build a positive framework of inner thoughts that will last your whole life."

The second thing you need, of course, are affirmations. Here are some hints about how to create and use them.

Keep it personal. Affirmations are for you and you alone, so examine your life for areas that could use improvement. Do you want to be more confident? Would you like to be less angry? Do you want to get along better with your co-workers? Pick one or two goals to start with, Dr. Jeffers says, and write down the rest to address later.

Make them short and sweet. Maybe you've decided that one of your goals is to stop worrying so much. Put your thoughts in positive form, state your affirmation in one sentence, and always form it in the present tense to make it more immediate. "I let go and trust" or "It's all working out perfectly" may work for you. Try saying your affirmations a few times to see if they click. "You can feel the tension releasing immediately if they're working," Dr. Jeffers says.

Pick affirmations that state the positive, says Dr. Jeffers. For example, say, "I am creating a successful career" instead of "I am not going to ruin my career."

Be realistic. Affirmations can help you achieve goals, but they are not magic incantations. "There's a fine line between *positive* thinking and *wishful* thinking," says Douglas Bloch, a Portland, Oregon–based counselor and lecturer and author of *Words That Heal: Affirmations and Meditations for Daily Living.* You'll probably have more success if you choose affirmations that deal with emotions, confidence, and self-esteem rather than material wealth, such as a new sports car.

That doesn't mean that you won't eventually get your dream car. Using affirmations correctly could help. An affirmation such as "I am confident and successful" could lead to "I am now ready to find a high-powered job" and maybe even to a real-life conversation along the lines of "I'll take that sports car now, Mr. Salesman."

Repeat, repeat, repeat. Say your affirmations daily. Dr. Jeffers suggests 20 to 30 repetitions per day. And make sure you say them out loud. "There's something about hearing them that makes them more powerful," she says. It's a good idea to set aside a regular time to say them, then add more whenever necessary.

Play it again—and again. In addition to your daily oral repetitions, try putting your affirmations on tape. Dr. Jeffers suggests playing them as you drift off to sleep and again right after you wake up. "Those are times when you're particularly likely to absorb the message," she says. Other good times are during a workout, when you're walking the dog, and while you're cooking dinner. If you don't like the sound of your unaccompanied voice, play some soothing background music while you record your affirmations.

Surprise yourself. Hide reminders in unexpected places. Write your affirmations on random days in your date book. Put them on a bookmark in a favorite novel. "Seeing your affirmations in odd places at odd times is a great way to reinforce the message," Dr. Jeffers says. "It's a jolt of positive energy."

Explore the spiritual. Affirmations work best when you tap into a higher power, Bloch says. "We derive strength from the feeling that we are not alone. It's comforting and freeing to ask for spiritual guidance," he says.

Try an affirmation like "I am truly blessed" or "Wherever I am, God is." If religious references make you uncomfortable, try looking inward toward what Dr. Jeffers calls your higher self. She suggests affirmations like "I trust in myself" or "I am one with the universe." She explains, "You don't have to believe there's a God. You just have to believe that you can reach a higher plane in your life through reflection and trust."

Don't stop. Affirmations are a long-term commitment, Dr. Jeffers says. Keep using them even when things are going well. "Otherwise, you may find yourself falling back into habits that pull you down," she says. "There can be a lot of negativity in the world, but the proper use of affirmations helps us to see the opportunity for growth in all things."

ALTRUISM

Helping Others to Help Yourself

What if research showed that one medicine could improve your overall health, reduce stress, relieve depression, and decrease your awareness of pain? Would you be interested?

That research is in. In a national survey of 3,000 Americans who took this medicine regularly, more than 95 percent said that they experienced heightened physical sensations, which for many led to the effects just described. The amazing prescription is altruism—helping other people—and it works.

The research also shows that there's a particular kind of altruism that over time boosts your health and happiness the most. It's not when you write a check for charity or when you take care of your family and friends (even though these bring fulfillment, too). The altruism that keeps you happier, healthier, and feeling younger is the kind that brings you into one-on-one contact with a stranger. Then the benefits bloom for both of you.

Helping a stranger in need begins to break down the sense of "them" versus "us," and that empathy is the key to experiencing the lasting euphoria and youthful energy that altruism brings, says Allan Luks, an attorney who heads New York City's Big Brother/Big Sister organization and who led the national volunteer survey, which he describes in his book, *The Healing Power of Doing Good.*

More than 20 volunteer organizations across the country participated in the survey. They were asked questions about the type and frequency of helping activities that they participated in, the state of their health, and their perceptions of the physical and emotional effects of helping.

The volunteers' responses suggest that people who are altruistic more frequently report better health and increased happiness, says Howard F. Andrews, Ph.D., an epidemiologist and senior staff associate in neurology at Columbia University College of Physicians and Surgeons in New York City. Dr. Andrews analyzed the data from Luks's research and concluded that those who help others often report significantly better health, including less depression, less pain, and even fewer visits to doctors.

Keep Your Spirit Young

"A miserly spirit is a dying spirit. My advice is to give. It's the only way of life that makes sense," says Millard Fuller, president and founder of Habitat for Humanity International in Americus, Georgia, the organization of volunteers who build houses for people in need.

Want to experience ageless spirit? Here's how.

Check out the possibilities. If you're at a loss as to where to begin, think of what you care about and head for the phone book, says Luks. "If you're concerned about a certain health problem or social cause, you'll often find a local nonprofit group in the telephone book," he says. "And many communities have a volunteer action center of some sort."

Find the right fit. You can also start by simply visualizing yourself in situations to see what feels like a good fit, Luks suggests. "Just imagine yourself: 'here I am tutoring for literacy' or 'here's me helping to paint a house.' Then, when you call an organization in the area you've chosen, say, 'Do you use volunteers? I'm thinking about volunteering. Can you send me some literature?' They'll be glad to hear from you."

Work one-on-one. Meeting and spending time with the person you're helping will have a much greater impact on you than if you limit your helping to less-personal tasks, such as collecting clothes or canned goods for the poor, says Luks. Of the volunteers he surveyed, only 5 percent of those who had one-to-one contact with the person they were helping did not report a feeling of euphoria. But people who never encountered those they helped were three times less likely to experience that youthful, buoyant feeling.

Join a team. It's even more effective to help strangers in the company of kindred spirits, such as through involvement with a supportive organization of volunteers. Dr. Andrews's analysis of the Luks data suggests that people who helped strangers through a group rather than on their own made significantly fewer visits to the doctor and reported more positive effects and lasting good feelings from helping.

Help regularly. Those warm holiday feelings inspire a desire in many of us to help people in need. But people who help frequently year-round will continue to experience the good feelings altruism brings the giver, Luks's national survey showed. So to reap its fullest benefits, make your volunteer activity a regular routine, Luks says.

Use your talents. When you use your own particular skills and knowledge to help others, the experience is even more satisfying, Luks says. He cites surveys that asked people who were already volunteering why they continued, and one of the reasons given frequently was that they were able to use their skills to do something useful. Using your own talents to help or support someone else gives you a particularly strong sense of usefulness, which in turn reduces stress, he says. If you're a lawyer, help at a free law clinic. If you can teach, you can tutor. If you can grow a vegetable, you can feed the hungry. The opportunities are limitless, Luks says.

Take a volunteer vacation. You can use your time off not only to rejuvenate your own spirit but also to help other people or rescue the environment. Habitat for Humanity International, for instance, will connect you with a nearby group working on housing for the poor, Fuller says. Write to them at 121 Habitat Street, Americus, GA 31709 for more information.

Or you could help to conserve endangered species, environments, or cultures as a member of the EarthCorps. EarthCorps volunteers join Earthwatch expeditions and assist scientists on research expeditions all over the globe. "You can help on one of 165 projects in 58 countries and 25 states," says Mary Blue Magruder, Earthwatch's director of public affairs. You can write to Earthwatch at P.O. Box 403 R.P., Watertown, MA 02272 for details.

The Healthy Helper

Although nothing beats the selfless experience of helping other people, you have to keep your own needs in mind, too, Luks says. Here are his tips on how to avoid disappointment and "volunteer burnout."

Help at your own pace. Start gradually and volunteer at a pace that's right for you, Luks says. If it starts to feel like a weary obligation, you're doing too much or you're in the wrong volunteer activity.

Don't fix everything. If you try to rescue the whole world, you'll set yourself up for disappointment, Luks says. Don't take on total responsibility for even one person or blame yourself for circumstances you can't control.

Do it together. A good way to deal with "beginner's nerves" and take the first step in getting involved is to pursue a volunteer activity as a family or with a friend, Luks says. You will strengthen your relationships as you each receive the emotional and health benefits of helping, he says.

Feel free to change your mind. If one situation or project isn't bringing you satisfaction and well-being, it's perfectly okay to look for another, Luks says. Nobody is indispensable, and you need to find the helping activity that's right for you. You'll know it's the right fit when you feel more energetic after a volunteering session than you did when you started.

ANTIOXIDANTS

The Best Defense Is
a Good Offense

It's one of life's great ironies. Oxygen—the glorious stuff that fills our lungs and keeps us alive—is involved in a process that can seriously hurt us.

To get the energy they need, your cells use oxygen to burn fuels such as glucose (blood sugar). In the process, some oxygen molecules may lose an electron. Those molecules then become what are known as free radicals, hell-bent on replacing their lost electrons by raiding the other molecules in the cell.

"Soon a chain reaction of electron theft begins that can produce widespread damage to the chemistry and function of the cell," says Denham Harman, M.D., Ph.D., professor emeritus of medicine and biochemistry at the University of Nebraska College of Medicine in Omaha.

Wrinkled skin, shrinking muscles, weak bones—many of the signs of growing old—could be due in part to this destructive oxidation process, the sum of millions of continuous free radical reactions. But of even greater concern to researchers is the notion that these free radicals are causing some of aging's most insidious diseases.

Atherosclerosis (hardening of the arteries), for instance, the leading cause of heart disease and stroke, is caused by the buildup of low-density lipoprotein (LDL) cholesterol, the so-called bad cholesterol. But it probably isn't until free radicals oxidize the LDL cholesterol that it assumes its potentially deadly form, according to Balz Frei, Ph.D., associate professor of medicine and biochemistry at the Boston University Medical Center.

Your body isn't entirely helpless when free radicals go on the warpath. In fact, it actually starts producing certain enzymes to combat the invaders. The problem is that it just doesn't produce enough to stop them all. It needs outside help—fast.

Enter dietary antioxidants—nutritional "scavengers" that patrol our bodies for free radicals, squelching the offending particles. "They actually render the free radicals harmless and head off the destructive chain reaction before damage can occur or spread out," Dr. Frei says.

Most researchers have focused their attentions on three antioxidant nutrients: vitamin C, vitamin E, and beta-carotene, a substance that the body converts to vitamin A. Study after study has shown that high doses of each of these nutrients result in low instances of many chronic diseases, including hypertension (high blood pressure), cataracts, and even certain types of cancer, such as oral, esophageal, stomach, lung, breast, and cervical cancer.

How Much Do You Need?

The National Research Council's Food and Nutrition Board has established the Recommended Dietary Allowances (RDAs) as guidelines for how much of each nutrient we need to consume each day to meet our basic health needs and prevent deficiency diseases. For women ages 25 to 50, the daily numbers are 60 milligrams of vitamin C, 8 milligrams alpha-tocopherol equivalents (or 12 international units) of vitamin E, and 800 micrograms retinol equivalents (or 4,000 international units) of vitamin A or 4.8 milligrams of beta-carotene. For men, it's 60 milligrams of C, 10 milligrams alpha-tocopherol equivalents (15 international units) of E, and 1,000 micrograms (or 5,000 international units) of A or 6 milligrams of beta-carotene.

"Four to five servings of fruits and vegetables per day should easily provide you with most if not all of the RDAs for the antioxidants as well as other important vitamins and minerals," says Diane Grabowski-Nepa, R.D., a nutrition educator at the Pritikin Longevity Center in Santa Monica, California.

That's fine for basic health, but in order to achieve the kind of disease-fighting results seen in scientific studies, you need to surpass the current RDAs. Most researchers believe that a combination of diet and supplements is the wisest choice. Note that nutritional supplements work best in conjunction with other healthy practices, such as eating low-fat, high-fiber meals, says Jeffrey Blumberg, Ph.D., professor of nutrition and associate director of the Jean Mayer USDA Human Nutrition Research Center on Aging at Tufts University in Boston. He recommends a daily intake of between 500 and 1,000 milligrams of vitamin C, between 100 and 400 international units of vitamin E, and between 6 and 30 milligrams of beta-carotene.

Getting Your Quota

Here's how you can best put antioxidants to work and prevent the harmful effects of free radicals.

Eat fewer calories. Digestion requires oxygen—lots of it. The more calories we consume, the more oxygen is required and the greater our chances for free radical formation. Cutting back on the amount we eat can trim our risk of oxidative damage, says Dr. Harman. That doesn't mean you should starve yourself or do anything to reduce your intake of the essential nutrients, he warns. Instead, focus on trimming those nonessential calories like desserts, candy, and soda from your diet.

Get some fresh air. Free radicals are also generated in the environment by industrial chemicals, heavy metals, fumes, car exhaust, air conditioning, and other airborne pollutants. While we can't escape all these man-made contaminants, anything that limits our exposure to them is beneficial, says Dr. Harman. For example, if you work in a factory or an office, you can take a walk at lunchtime to briefly get away from impurities that may be circulating around your workplace. Open windows. Or use a commercial air-purifying device.

Snuff out the cigarettes. Cigarette smoke contributes huge amounts of free radicals with every puff. Antioxidants can prevent much of the oxidative damage caused by smoking, says Dr. Frei. But if you avoid the habit in the first place, those antioxidants will be available to fight free radicals elsewhere in the body.

Go easy on the hard stuff. The occasional cocktail isn't going to cause any harm and may actually lower your risk of heart disease, but frequent alcohol consumption can increase the number of free radicals in the body, says Dr. Frei. Not only that, but people with alcoholism show reduced levels of antioxidants in their systems. According to a study at the King's College School of Medicine and Dentistry in London, alcoholic patients showed significantly lower levels of vitamin E and beta-carotene, which coincided respectively with higher incidences of cirrhosis and liver damage.

Don't overdo your workouts. When it comes to exercise, remember the adage "train, don't strain." As beneficial as exercise is to your health, the extra oxygen you take in whenever you work out subjects muscles and other tissues to additional oxidative damage. Pushing the body beyond its limits can lead to an overproduction of free radicals, and that can have a devastating effect on the way you look and feel. "This may be why athletes who overtrain find that their performance suffers or they become sick," says Robert R. Jenkins, Ph.D., professor of biology at Ithaca College in New York.

Does this mean you shouldn't exercise? Absolutely not. Most doctors and scientists believe that any oxidative damage is minimal with normal exercise and is offset by the added benefits that exercise provides. According to a British study of endurance runners, regular, nonexhaustive exercise enhances the levels of some antioxidant enzymes in the blood. And a study conducted at the Washington University School of Medicine in St. Louis found that high doses of vitamin C, vitamin E, and beta-carotene, while not preventing the body from undergoing any exercise-induced oxidative stress, do seem to lower the signs of oxidative damage in the body.

Regular, moderate exercise seems to strike the perfect balance, says Dr. Harman. And no matter what, keep up your intake of antioxidant vitamins.

BREAST CARE

Keeping Your Breasts Firm and Healthy

You turn to the right and look at your breasts sideways in the mirror. You turn to the front, lift your arms over your head, and check again. Then you turn to the left and check one more time. What are you looking for?

Two things: the sags and stretch marks that suggest you're beginning to age and any lumps, bumps, dimples, or changes that may signal the presence of cancer.

While no one welcomes the signs of aging, what women fear most is breast cancer. And for good reason—it's the most common type of cancer that women get. And most breast cancer is found by women themselves—not by a doctor or a mammogram—when they notice that something doesn't look or feel right. Yet 80 percent of women say that they don't do breast self-examinations on a regular basis.

Breast cancer is a major health threat to any woman over 30, says Sondra Lynne Carter, M.D., a gynecologist in private practice in New York City. And the threat escalates with every year.

The Breast Self-Exam

Good breast care begins with learning when and how to do a breast self-exam. Doctors agree that a self-exam should be done the first week after your period every month. Your goal is twofold: one, to become so familiar with the normal ridges, lumps, and bumps in your breasts that anything out of the ordinary will be very apparent; and, two, to detect any lump (about one-half inch in size, for example) that suddenly appears, stays in the same place, and remains for one or two cycles.

Here's how doctors suggest you make a breast exam as accurate as possible.

Stretch first. Before you start, stretch your arms over your head and look in the mirror to see if there are any obvious changes in your breasts. Look for something major: dimpling that you've never noticed before or a nipple that has suddenly inverted, developed eczema, or has a discharge that isn't the result of being squeezed. Put your hands on your hips, push your shoulders back, and look for changes again. Then push your shoulders forward, contracting your chest muscles. Any dimpling should be obvious in this position.

Choose a search strategy. There are several different ways to do the breast exam itself: You can use the nipple as a focal point and feel for lumps along imaginary lines radiating out from the nipple all the way up to the collarbone and down to the brassiere line; you can use the nipple as a center and keep circling it with your fingers in ever-larger circles; or you can simply imagine a grid placed over your breast and examine it in up-to-the-collarbone and down-to-the-bra-line strips.

Whichever method you choose, put the hand on the side you want to examine behind your head before you start. This shifts any breast tissue that's under your armpit over to the chest wall where you can check it thoroughly.

The Anti-Cancer Lifestyle

Women who reduce the amount of estrogen circulating throughout their bodies may significantly reduce their risk of developing breast cancer. And that includes women who have a family history of the disease. Which strategies are best? Here's what doctors suggest.

Lower the fat. A study at Tufts University School of Medicine in Boston compared women who ate a diet that got 40 percent of its calories from fat with women who got only 21 percent of their calories from fat. The result? Premenopausal women in the higher-fat group had blood levels of estrogen that were 30 to 75 percent higher. Postmenopausal women who ate the higher-fat diet had estrogen levels that were 300 percent higher.

Eat plant fiber. Animal studies indicate that phytoestrogens in plants may be able to prevent the estrogens circulating in your body from causing breast cancer. Good sources of phytoestrogens include soy products, alfalfa sprouts, apples, barley, oats, and peas.

Nosh on veggies. In the Harvard University's Nurses' Health Study, which studied nearly 90,000 women in Boston, researchers found that those who ate two or three servings of vegetables a day had a 17 percent reduced risk of breast cancer compared with those who ate less than one full serving per day. Scientists suspect that it may have something to do with the presence of vitamin C and beta-carotene, antioxidants believed to block cancer-causing substances produced by the body's normal metabolic process.

Avoid midcycle drinking. A study at the National Cancer Institute found that just two mixed drinks a day between days 12 and 15 of a woman's menstrual cycle elevate estrogen levels anywhere from 21 to 31 percent.

Beating Breast Sag

Although good breast care primarily means keeping your breasts healthy, for some women it also means keeping their breasts smooth and firm. Fortunately, there are several ways to prevent—and sometimes reverse—both sag and stretch marks.

Think weights. "There's no way I know of to build up the breast's fatty tissue," says Dr. Carter. "But you can build up the pectoralis muscles underlying the fatty tissues so that you get the same effect." To prevent or reduce sag, get a couple of two-pound weights—no heavier—and work those muscles five times a week, she says.

With a weight in each hand, extend your arms sideways and do 15 small, backward circles about a foot in diameter. Widen the circles slightly and do another 15, then widen them again and repeat. Slowly work your way up to 20 circles for each repetition.

Roll your shoulders. Put your weights aside and with your arms hanging at your sides, roll your shoulders backward, down, and forward in a circular motion 15 to 20 times, says Dr. Carter. Do it five days a week.

Hit the deck. "Start off trying to do 10 push-ups and work your way up to 20," says Dr. Carter. It may take up to six months, but you're more likely to do them regularly if you add one push-up at a time. Just get on your hands and knees, raise your feet six inches off the floor, and lower your upper body to within an inch of the floor. Do these five days a week.

Get some support. Wearing a bra is a good way to prevent sagging, says Albert M. Kligman, M.D., professor of dermatology at the

University of Pennsylvania School of Medicine in Philadelphia. Get a style that has great support and allows minimal bounce. And wear it all day, not just when you work out.

Shrink the stretch marks. If you've just had a baby and the stretch marks on the top and sides of your breasts are red and inflamed, you can treat them with daily applications of tretinoin (Retin-A), says Dr. Kligman. Talk to your doctor about getting a prescription. Retin-A not only tightens the stretched skin but may also build a new super-structure under the skin to help firm it.

Talk to your doctor about HRT. Hormone replacement therapy, or HRT, can halt breast sagging that occurs after menopause by helping to keep breast fibers from further degenerating, doctors say. It won't turn the clock back to your twenties, but it will keep your breasts from sagging more.

CONFIDENCE AND SELF-ESTEEM

Be Your Own Best Friend

Do you think highly of yourself, or do you see yourself as over the hill and going headlong into the valley of antiquity? Confidence and self-esteem really are matters not of age or appearance but of attitude. And they produce some very youth-engendering results.

For starters, they do wonders for your mind. They provide a buffer against anxiety and relieve feelings of guilt, hopelessness, and inadequacy. They give us the courage to fulfill our dreams. Best of all, confidence and self-esteem are self-perpetuating, giving us the power not only to survive but also to embrace life.

Hold Your Head High

If you feel that your confidence and self-esteem could use a boost, that's probably a sign that they could. Here's what the experts recommend.

Shape up. In one study at the State University of New York College at Brockport, 57 people were divided into two groups: One group lifted weights for 16 weeks, while the other group completed a physical education theory course. Guess which group wound up with the lifted spirits?

Merrill J. Melnick, Ph.D., the sports sociologist who led the study, explains why the exercise group fared so much better: "You may see yourself as inferior if you're unhappy with your physical self." By building a little muscle and losing a little fat, he says, you can improve your feelings about your body and about yourself.

Gag your internal critic. People with low self-esteem tend to hear little voices in their heads that say, "You can't," "You're weak," "You're worthless." Whenever your critical inner voice begins putting you down, silence it immediately, says Bonnie Jacobson, Ph.D., director of the Institute for Psychological Change in New York City. Counter its arguments with assertions to the contrary. Tell yourself over and over that you are strong, capable, and worthy, until the voice goes away. If unhappy thoughts still get the better of you, schedule a 30-minute worry session to get them out of your system; then get on with enjoying life.

Take a personal inventory. "Instead of dwelling on our shortcomings, we need to draw satisfaction from the things we have and can do well," says Stanley Teitelbaum, Ph.D., a clinical psychologist in private practice in New York City. To do this, list all your achievements, activities, positive traits, and strengths on one side of a piece of paper. Then list your weaknesses, negative traits, and things you wish you could change on the other side. You may be surprised to learn just how much is going in your favor—and this alone can make you feel remarkably good. For long-term confidence and self-esteem, accentuate the positives.

Set up a hierarchy of goals. "Reaching for a goal is great, but you must learn to crawl before you can walk," says Thomas Tutko, Ph.D., professor of psychology at San Jose State University in California. Suppose you have a goal of bowling a 300 game. A worthy goal, but it's somewhat unrealistic if your average is, say, 58. Instead of shooting for your ultimate goal, concentrate on reaching plateaus. "Find success on one level first, then try to transfer it up to the next," he says.

Specialize in something. Are you a jack of all trades and master of none? Spreading yourself too thin only sets you up for disappointment, says Dr. Tutko. Find two or three things in life that you really enjoy and focus most of your energies on them. It's better to be successful at a few things than to fail at many.

Pursue what you love. The easiest way to lose faith in yourself is to get trapped doing something that you dislike or that others tell you "you're supposed to do," says Dr. Tutko. Rather than wallow in a career or activity that makes you miserable or that you attempt halfheartedly, seek out those things that really turn you on and pursue them with gusto. You're more likely to do them well, which will have a positive effect on your psyche.

Be of service. Lending your time and talents to help your community or people in need boosts confidence and self-esteem in many ways, says Dr. Jacobson. Foremost, it gives you a wonderful feeling of accomplishment and reinforces your belief that you are worthwhile.

Seek out positive people. The last thing you need in your life when your self-confidence is flagging is people who criticize or find fault with you. Instead, you should surround yourself with people who look for the good in you. Invariably, those are people who themselves have high levels of confidence and self-esteem. "People with high self-esteem and confidence aren't quick to judge or put down others," says Dr. Jacobson. "They have a lot of love and encouragement to give, and their attitudes toward life can rub off on you."

Reward yourself. Stroke your confidence and self-esteem by doing something nice for yourself whenever you do something well, says Dr. Tutko. Congratulate yourself or treat yourself to a little gift. This reinforces your faith in yourself and gives the value of your accomplishment more weight.

Be *your* best, not *the* best. Competitive sports are a great way to enhance your confidence and self-esteem. But if you consider beating opponents and winning trophies the only measures of success, your confidence and self-esteem are already on shaky ground. "Playing sports can be fantastic, but only if you do it for the sheer love of it and for the exploration of being the best you possibly can," says Dr. Tutko.

Don't fear failure. View failure not as an evil but as an opportunity for a new success, says Daniel Wegner, Ph.D., professor of psychology at the University of Virginia in Charlottesville. "Life is a trial-and-error process, and we don't make any progress if we don't take chances in the face of failure," he says. "In the grand scheme of things, most of the actual 'failures' we will experience are not nearly as harmful as the damage we do to ourselves when we obsess and worry about our failures yet to come."

FIBER

Staying Young Inside and Out

Mom always knew best. Like when she had you start your day with oatmeal. And when she packed your lunch with carrots and apples—what she used to call roughage.

Today, science has proven what Mom always said: There's something special about fruits, vegetables, and grains that really does a body good. And roughage is what nutritionists now call dietary fiber, one of the simplest and most potent weapons we have in our age-erasing arsenal.

Fiber is a front-line warrior in the battle against heart disease, breast and other cancers, atherosclerosis, high cholesterol, high blood pressure, constipation, digestive problems, diabetes, and even overweight. Get enough fiber and your body will be healthier and run like a well-oiled machine.

But most people don't get enough. "The recommended intake is at least 20 to 35 grams of fiber every day," says Diane Grabowski-Nepa, R.D., a nutrition educator at the Pritikin Longevity Center in Santa Monica, California. "Most Americans, however, only consume about one-third of that total."

Fiber is a complex mixture of indigestible substances that make up the structural material of plants. It has very few calories and provides little food energy to the body. Fiber works its magic by carrying the bad stuff—like cholesterol, bile acids, and other toxins—

out of your system. And it comes in two basic forms: soluble, which dissolves in water, and insoluble, which doesn't. Most plant foods contain both types, although certain foods are richer in one or the other.

The coarser insoluble fibers really live up to the word *roughage.* "They literally scour you out," says David Jenkins, M.D., Ph.D., director of the Clinical Nutrition and Risk Factor Modification Center at St. Michael's Hospital at the University of Toronto. Insoluble fiber also makes a natural remedy for constipation, irritable bowel syndrome, diverticulosis, and hemorrhoids.

Soluble fibers act differently. Inside the body, they become gummy and sticky. As they move through the digestive tract, they pick up bile acids and other toxins, then haul them out of the body.

Fiber plays a vital role in the offensive against heart disease and atherosclerosis. Studies have shown that a diet high in soluble fiber reduces blood levels of low-density lipoprotein (LDL) cholesterol, the so-called bad cholesterol. A study by Dr. Jenkins found that high intakes of soluble fiber continued to lower cholesterol even after dietary reductions of fat and cholesterol had been achieved.

One surefire way to get a heap of fiber into your diet is by eating bran, the coarse outer layers of oats, wheat, rice, and corn that contain the highest concentrations of fiber.

Oat bran has received the most public attention in recent years. "What sets oat bran apart from other brans is that it is extremely high in a fiber called beta-glucan," says bran researcher Michael H. Davidson, M.D., medical director of the Chicago Center for Clinical Research at Rush-Presbyterian–St. Luke's Hospital. "Beta-glucan appears to be far more effective than other soluble fibers in lowering blood cholesterol levels."

Just two ounces of oat bran per day (a medium bowl) is enough to lower your LDL cholesterol 10 to 15 percent. The catch is that you have to eat oat bran daily; otherwise, your cholesterol levels will creep back up.

Wheat bran is jam-packed with insoluble fiber, so it's the bran of choice for people with digestive problems. This is the most common bran, found in most bran breakfast cereals and all whole-wheat products. Rice, oat, and corn bran are high in both soluble and insoluble fiber. Probably the best plan is to get a smattering of each for healthy variety.

Getting your fill of bran is as easy as eating bran breakfast cereal, a bran muffin, or whole-grain bread. But make sure you're always getting the goodness of the bran. "Refined grain products like white rice, white bread, and most flour have had the fiber-rich bran removed in the milling process," says Grabowski-Nepa. "Instant oatmeal, for example, has a lot less fiber than whole oats or pure oat bran."

Adding Fiber to Your Life

Making the commitment to a high-fiber diet is relatively easy. Here are some tips.

Ease into it. As great as fiber is, eating too much, too fast can have some nasty side effects, including gas, bloating, diarrhea, and cramps, says Dr. Jenkins. Start off your first week by increasing your intake by about five grams a day. Then take about a month to work up to the recommended level. From there, if your doctor says it's okay and if you feel no ill effects, you can increase your intake even more.

Don't dry out. We all know that a high-fiber diet helps constipation, but if you don't get enough water, it can actually have an opposite effect, says Dr. Jenkins. Drink 8 to 10 glasses of water a day to prevent constipation.

Vary your sources. Doctors aren't certain what ratio of soluble to insoluble fiber you should use when choosing your daily 20 to 35 grams, says Dr. Jenkins, so it's probably wise to get equal doses of each. The best strategy is to eat a wide variety of fiber-rich foods throughout the day.

Go for the green. "Don't forget your fresh fruits and vegetables," advises Grabowski-Nepa. Legumes, beans, peas, salads, and fruits can add a whole lot of the much-needed fiber to your diet. For some extra fiber, select fruits that have edible seeds, such as strawberries and kiwis.

Add a few sprinkles. "Fiber is easy to obtain in your diet if you include whole foods such as whole-wheat bread, beans, peas, and fresh fruits and vegetables," says Grabowski-Nepa. But for additional fiber, pick up a box of oat bran and sprinkle it on yogurt, ice cream, fruit, breakfast cereal, and salads. Use it in place of bread crumbs in meat loaf or stuffings or as a thickener for soups, stews, and sauces. Or substitute oat bran for some of the white flour in baked goods.

Read labels carefully. Don't assume that a product with the words *fiber, bran,* or *oats* in its title necessarily has the fiber content you're looking for. Always check the nutritional information on the box or bag to see just how much fiber is available in each serving. "Also, look for the word *whole* preceding *grain* on the ingredient list," suggests Grabowski-Nepa. "This way you know that nothing has been removed, and you are sure to get the full benefit of the bran."

Avoid fiber pills. Fiber pills and drink mixes are a quick way to get more fiber, but most professionals don't recommend them, says Grabowski-Nepa. They're expensive, and it takes several pills and drinks to equal the fiber content of a piece of fruit. Your best bet is to meet your fiber requirements by eating foods that are naturally rich in fiber.

Go whole. Slight changes in the way you eat can infuse your diet with fiber, says Grabowski-Nepa. Instead of your morning glass of orange juice, try eating a whole piece of fruit since almost all the fiber gets left behind in the juicing process. Serve whole brown rice instead of white. And if you like meat and potatoes, substitute a baked potato with the skin in place of mashed spuds.

FLUIDS

Life's Liquid Assets

It's the most abundant compound on Earth. A vital nutrient. And a powerful age-erasing ally. What is it? Water. A substance so simple, so common that it's easy to overlook its importance.

Present in every cell and tissue, water plays a vital role in almost every biological process. It transports nutrients throughout the body and carries harmful toxins and waste products out. It regulates body temperature. And it lubricates our joints and organs.

Because water does so much, you need a constant fresh supply. "Water needs to continuously flow in, through, and out of the body," says Diane Grabowski-Nepa, R.D., a nutrition educator with the Pritikin Longevity Center in Santa Monica, California. "It's a key ingredient if you want to look, feel, and perform at your very best."

Fill 'Er Up

When experts recommend consuming six to eight eight-ounce glasses of liquid a day, that can mean water, juice, broths, or other beverages. "A good rule is to try to drink about one-half ounce for each pound of body weight," says Grabowski-Nepa. You'll need more if you're dieting, living in a hot or dry environment, or sick with fever, vomiting, or diarrhea, all of which can rob your body of its fluids.

It's fairly simple to keep up your fluid intake. Here's how.

Greet the day with a glass. As you slept, your body went for hours without water. So pour yourself a glass after you wake up, says

Grabowski-Nepa. Don't rely on your morning coffee, which can be dehydrating because it's a diuretic.

Keep it up. Don't try to guzzle your entire daily intake at once. You'll feel like you're bursting at the seams and simply excrete more, says Grabowski-Nepa. Instead, take frequent water breaks—about one every hour or two—so you're constantly hydrated. Drink even more if it's hot or humid or if your eyes, mouth, or skin feels dry.

Eat regularly. Much of your daily fluid intake comes during meals. Eat plenty of water-rich foods such as fruits and vegetables and always have a glass of water or another beverage with your meal, says Grabowski-Nepa.

Skip alcohol and caffeine. Booze, beer, coffee, tea, and colas are diuretics—that is, they encourage fluid excretion. These beverages may quench your thirst initially, but they ultimately draw fluids out of your body, says Grabowski-Nepa.

Avoid water-sapping foods. Salty foods can dry you out, says Grabowski-Nepa. If you must have them, limit your intake and make sure you drink plenty of fluids.

Watch those laxatives. Frequent use can draw an enormous amount of water from the body and disrupt the normal function of your digestive and elimination systems. You shouldn't take them regularly unless you're under a doctor's care, Grabowski-Nepa says.

Don't toss the pulp. Home juicing machines provide a great means for getting your daily fluids, says Grabowski-Nepa. But some completely separate the juice from the fruit or vegetable pulp, the part that contains the greatest concentration of fiber, nutrients, and water. Put some of that pulp into your glass.

Managing Exercise and Fluids

We can sweat away two quarts an hour when we exercise or play sports, especially if it's extremely hot and humid, says Miriam E. Nelson, Ph.D., a research scientist and exercise physiologist in the Human Physiology Laboratory at the Jean Mayer USDA Human Nutrition Research Center on Aging at Tufts University in Boston. That's why active people need to pay attention to their fluid needs. Keep these tips in mind.

Drink before, during, and after. Drink 8 to 20 ounces of water an hour before your workout, says Dr. Nelson. "Body size and ambient temperature affect the amount of water that you should drink." Don't overdose on water, however, as this will result in poor performance, she warns. Symptoms of too much water intake include an uncomfortable bloated feeling and stomach cramps. As you exercise, try to drink up to one-half to three-quarters cup of water every 10 minutes. Afterward, drink as much as you need to quench your thirst.

Hop on a scale. If you weigh yourself before and after you exercise, you'll find out how much water you lost. For every half-pound you lose, drink eight fluid ounces.

Go beyond thirst. Even if your immediate thirst feels quenched, your body's fluid reserves may not be adequately refilled, says Dr. Nelson. Play it safe and take a few additional sips. A few minutes later, drink some more. Continue for about an hour afterward.

Cool it. Cool water will lower your body temperature faster than warmer water. It's also dispersed much faster to the parched tissues of the body, Dr. Nelson says.

Adjust to your environment. If you come out of an air-conditioned building on a hot day and immediately try jogging five miles, the shock to your system will draw more water from your body than if you slowly accustom yourself to the outdoor heat, Dr. Nelson says.

Block the sun. Direct sunlight on a hot summer day will dry you like a prune, says Dr. Nelson. If you exercise in the heat and sun, wear a hat and light, loose-fitting clothing that breathes and lets in cool air. "If you feel dizzy or disoriented, stop exercising immediately," she warns. Find some shade and fluids to help lower your body temperature.

Ease into it. If you haven't been exercising, don't try to take on an advanced exercise program. Because you'll have to exert yourself more, you'll sweat more than someone who is in better shape. To avoid dehydration risk, start your workout program slowly, get used to exercising, and gradually increase the intensity, says Dr. Nelson.

Use sports drinks sparingly. Sports drinks, which are rich in the electrolytes that we lose when we exercise, are often touted for their replenishing abilities, but they are no more effective than water, according to Dr. Nelson. The only time these drinks have an advantage over water is if you have just come off an extremely draining workout, such as a marathon. Then you may need an immediate electrolyte boost.

FRIENDSHIPS

They're Good for Life

Friendship has a profound effect on your physical well-being," says Eugene Kennedy, Ph.D., professor of psychology at Loyola University of Chicago. "Having good relationships improves health and lifts depression. You don't necessarily need drugs or medical treatment to accomplish this—just friends," he says. And perhaps one of the greatest health benefits of friendship is the youthfulness of extended life—the addition of years of enjoyment and satisfaction.

One of the first studies linking social relationships and longevity took place in Alameda County, California. Researchers there found that over a nine-year period, the people with the strongest social and community ties were the least likely to die. Not surprisingly, the most isolated people had the highest death rates.

Redford B. Williams, M.D., professor of psychiatry and director of the Behavioral Research Center at Duke University Medical Center in Durham, North Carolina, sees a definite connection between friendship and longevity. His team studied 1,368 heart disease patients for nine years. "What we found," says Dr. Williams, "was that those patients with neither a spouse nor a close friend were three times more likely to die than those involved in a caring relationship."

Women tend to have more intimate friendships than men do. "Women are more emotional and more willing to express emotional needs. When they feel the need to meet new people or just to talk, they're much more likely to approach someone," says Michael Cunningham, Ph.D., professor of psychology at the University of Louisville in Kentucky. Men's friendships are traditionally with people they meet at work. Work offers a common interest to base a friendship on, but the problem with work relationships is they tend to last only as long as the job does.

Among both sexes, many people have difficulty developing relationships because they lack certain relationship-building skills. Fortunately, it's never too late to start learning them.

You Reap What You Sow

Friends don't spring up like wildflowers. They have to be cultivated like roses. And like roses, they'll keep blooming and growing as long as you nourish them. Here are some tips for growing a garden of friends—and reaping the age-erasing benefits of love and friendship.

Be a friend for life. Friendships don't happen overnight. They require exchanges of trust and confidence that can only develop over time. You have to maintain and nourish your friends by showing genuine, continuing interest in them. Don't just say, "How are you?" Say it and really listen to the response. And then tell them how you are.

Try new activities. Often you attract friends to the extent that you are doing things they are interested in, says Dr. Cunningham. The message: "Be willing to try new activities that will put you in contact with people who might turn out to be good friends," he says.

Be open and be real. "Friendship depends on sharing and responding to each other," says Dr. Kennedy. "There's no formula for making friends. The real requirement is just being yourself and showing who you are to someone else."

Many people have the idea that revealing themselves is a tremendous risk and that they might face ridicule, says Arthur Wassmer, Ph.D., a psychologist in private practice in Kirkland, Washington, and author of *Making Contact*. This feeling usually comes from low self-esteem and makes some believe that they aren't worthy of sharing their feelings with others, he says. In reality, he adds, you're almost never going to get a bad response from someone when you try to be genuine and open with something personal.

Make yourself likable. Likability is a talent. And like any talent, it can be honed, says Dr. Wassmer. To increase your odds of being liked when meeting strangers, break the ice with questions like "Where are you from?" and "Are you enjoying the party?" Be an active listener. Reveal your feelings and experiences. And be sure to hand out compliments.

Ask for what you need. Just because you tell someone your problems doesn't mean that you'll get the emotional support you need, according to Dr. Cunningham. If you want advice, say so. If you want acceptance and sympathy, let your friend know that, too.

Project friendly body language. In his work with shy people, Dr. Wassmer learned that the way you move is just as important as what you say when you're trying to make friends. He offers these tips for presenting yourself in a social situation so you'll appear open and inviting. Smile. Practice open posture (meaning, for instance, don't cross your arms). Lean toward people, not away from them. Occasionally, give them a light touch on the shoulder or arm. Make eye contact. And nod in agreement as you converse.

Find sympathetic people. It's a Catch-22, but people who are lonely and needy have the most trouble making friends. Dr. Cunningham says that people develop "social allergies" to needy people and become wary and irritated with them. That's why it helps to look for friends among people who understand what you're going through. If you're a grieving widow or a recovering addict or if you suffer from any number of alienating problems, look into the self-help or 12-step groups in your area. These groups can help an isolated person deal with problems and eventually become less needy and thus more attractive to others.

Have all types of buddies. Try having simple nonsexual friendships with members of the opposite sex whom you like. Sometimes women appreciate their men friends because they provide the male point of view, and it can be useful to hear the male angle once in a while. Men, on the other hand, often feel more comfortable expressing their feelings to a woman than to another man.

Find a furry friend. Numerous studies have shown that pets are good for health and longevity. Although all sorts of companion animals have been shown to have therapeutic effects, dogs seem to have an edge, particularly in providing comfort and support to older people. But whether you decide to walk a dog, stroke a cat, or talk to a canary, you'll get love, ease stress, and bolster your heart health.

Reach out and fax someone. These days, people are so busy that it can be difficult to find time for friends. But there are always telephones, faxes, e-mail, and old-fashioned letters. You don't have to have constant direct contact to maintain a good friendship.

Don't put all your eggs in one basket. It can be dangerous to rely on one person for all of your emotional support, whether it's a friend or a spouse. What if your only friend gets tired of listening to you? Or what if your spouse is no longer there? You'll suddenly be isolated, and you will probably feel a lot older in a short period of time. It's wiser to spread your emotional needs among various people.

GOALS

Your Road Map to Vitality

Goals can help you keep your mind and body in peak condition, says Dennis Gersten, M.D., a psychiatrist in private practice in San Diego and publisher of *Atlantis: The Imagery Newsletter.* "If you don't have goals, what happens? You won't be motivated to maintain your health and keep up your body," he says. "Your life won't have meaning, and you won't feel complete. So having goals makes you whole spiritually, physically, and emotionally. And being whole can make you healthier and relieve stress."

Goals also help prevent boredom, and that's important because boredom can put you at higher risk for disease, says Howard Friedman, Ph.D., professor of psychology and community medicine at the University of California, Riverside, and author of *The Self-Healing Personality.*

Charting Your Strategy

Your goals don't need to be grandiose or spectacular to energize you, says Dr. Gersten. But do make the effort to see that they're carefully shaped so it's more likely that your dreams will be transformed into reality. Here's how to reach for the stars.

Write 'em down. Committing your goals to paper will make them more tangible to you, says Dr. Friedman. Keep your list in a conspicuous place and check off your goals as you achieve them. Be sure to include a mixture of easy goals that will encourage you, such as reading the newspaper every day, and several more difficult ones that will challenge you, like increasing your productivity at work 10 percent.

Do first things first. After you list your goals, decide which ones are most important to you and start working on them. "People often do the least important things first, and the things that are really important to them never get done," Dr. Friedman says.

Be picky. Try not to spread yourself too thin. If you have more goals than you can realistically accomplish, you'll drain your energy and feel discouraged and depressed. It's better to have one or two well-defined goals that are meaningful to you than a dozen less important ones, Dr. Friedman says.

Love your goal. Choose goals that you feel passionate about so that you'll be more likely to follow through on them, Dr. Gersten says. If you start collecting stamps but your heart really isn't in it, you're probably not going to stick with it. But if you're a tennis fan, odds are that you'll be more successful if you start collecting tennis memorabilia.

Be real. Goals not only need to be specific, they should be realistic, says Marilee C. Goldberg, Ph.D., a psychotherapist in private practice in Lambertville, New Jersey, who specializes in cognitive and behavior therapy. If you say you're never going to watch television again, that's probably not realistic because goals that include absolute words like *always* or *never* seldom are achievable. A more specific and reasonable goal might be to limit your viewing to no more than two hours each evening.

Make it good for you. A goal that is torturous to achieve or jeopardizes your health isn't worthwhile. "Some people will say, 'I'll kill myself to do this thing.' You have to take your well-being into account no matter what your goal is. So if you want to plant a garden but you have a sore back, forcing yourself to get down on your knees and do it is a poor idea. If it's really that important to you, ask a friend or pay someone to do it," says Dr. Goldberg.

Set deadlines. Without time lines to nudge us along, many of us would never reach our goals. "Setting a deadline doesn't mean that you're bad if you don't make it," Dr. Goldberg says. "But a deadline does give you a point in time to shoot for. Then if you haven't accomplished everything you'd planned when time is up, forgive yourself, reevaluate your plan, and reset your time line."

Divide and conquer. Chopping your goal down into several intermediate steps will make it seem less overwhelming and more achievable, Dr. Goldberg says. If you want to set aside $2,500 over the next two years for a trip to England, you're probably going to have a harder time saving the money if you set your sights on getting the whole amount than if you find ways to save $3.50 a day or $24 a week.

Involve your friends. If you tell a friend about your goal or, better yet, get him to help you work on it, you'll be more motivated to stick to it, Dr. Friedman says.

Find an idol. If someone you admire has achieved a goal similar to yours, use that person for inspiration, Dr. Gersten says. Put his picture or quotes in a prominent place such as your desk or refrigerator. Take a moment each day to imagine the thrill of achieving what he did.

But don't compete. You should learn from the success of others, but you shouldn't set out to outdo them. If you're a songwriter, for example, you should study the works of the great pop artists, but you shouldn't feel as if you need to sell more recordings than Madonna to be a success. "You'll be less stressed and more creative if you try to be the best that you can be, rather than trying to be the best in the world," Dr. Gersten says.

Let go of your ego. Prepare yourself for rejection and criticism. In fact, you should welcome it because criticism can help you focus your goal. "When you begin working on a goal that is important to you, you should put your ego aside and let people chop your work up," Dr. Gersten says. "If you want to successfully reach your goal, you have to open yourself up to criticism."

Forget perfection. If you think that you have to do something perfectly, you'll probably never achieve your goals—all you'll end up doing is discouraging yourself. "You want to do your very best, but your goal shouldn't be perfection," Dr. Gersten says.

Keep your perspective. Goals are fine, but if they interfere with your family or social life, you could be headed for trouble, according to Brian Little, Ph.D., professor of psychology at Carleton University in Ottawa, Ontario.

Envision success. Imagine that you've already achieved your goal and that people are praising your effort. It may motivate you to accomplish the goal and do it well. "I imagine the book that I'm writing is at the top of the *New York Times* best-seller list, and that makes me want to create the best book that I can," Dr. Gersten says.

Treat yourself. Give yourself rewards such as a new compact disc, baseball tickets, or some nonfat frozen yogurt when you complete a goal, no matter how small, Dr. Goldberg suggests. It serves as an incentive to set and accomplish new tasks. And don't forget to give yourself a pat on the back.

Update your goals. "It's important to reassess your goals every six months because circumstances may have changed, and some goals may not fit your needs anymore," Dr. Goldberg says. If that's the case, don't hang on to it. Let it fade away and then choose something else that is important to you now.

HORMONE REPLACEMENT THERAPY

A *Midlife Option*

You've made a lot of health decisions in your lifetime. Now with menopause ahead, you face another. And this time, it feels like a real biggie. You keep mulling over the question: "Should I take hormone replacement therapy?"

Millions of baby boomers are asking themselves the same thing. It's estimated that more women than ever—from 40 to 50 million—will enter menopause during the next two decades.

We've all heard about the possible difficulties of menopause: hot flashes and night sweats, vaginal dryness and skin changes, and increased risk for heart disease and osteoporosis once menopause has passed. We've also heard about hormone replacement therapy as a means to combat these aging effects.

Whether to take hormone replacement therapy is often one of the first questions women have about menopause, says Joan Borton, a licensed mental health counselor in private practice in Rockport, Massachusetts, and author of *Drawing from the Women's Well: Reflections on the Life Passage of Menopause.*

The choice is difficult because there are both benefits and risks to taking hormone replacement therapy, or HRT. Women often find themselves trying to weigh the pros (HRT can relieve hot flashes and vaginal dryness, protect against heart disease and osteoporosis, and maintain youthful skin and hair) against the cons (women worry that it may increase their risk for breast cancer, uterine cancer, and gallstones). HRT also causes women to start having their periods again, which some view as an inconvenience. Most experts agree that the decision is an individual one.

HRT is a formulation of hormones designed to restore a woman's natural hormone levels. In the years preceding menopause, estrogen levels steadily decline. Then after ovulation stops and a woman has her last period, estrogen levels plunge even further.

Estrogen plays a vital role in maintaining tissues and organs throughout a woman's body. When estrogen levels dip low during menopause, there can be vaginal dryness, skin wrinkling, and deterioration in bone mass and strength. Estrogen also affects functions such as metabolism and body temperature regulation. When estrogen levels decline, a woman's cholesterol can rise, placing her at increased risk for heart disease. Her body's internal thermometer can also be thrown off-kilter, thus causing hot flashes and night sweats.

Years ago, hormone formulations contained just estrogen and were called estrogen replacement therapy, or ERT. When those caused problems, such as promoting uterine cancer, they were redesigned to lower the estrogen content and add a synthetic form of the hormone progesterone called progestin. It's that combination of estrogen and progestin that's known as HRT.

Hot flashes and vaginal dryness are the two main symptoms that send a woman to her doctor about menopause and HRT. Experts say that HRT is highly effective against hot flashes. Vaginal dryness also responds to HRT because the tissue of the vagina contains estrogen receptors. When estrogen declines, the linings of the vagina and uterus thin, and vaginal dryness results.

A woman's skin may also have estrogen receptors, so low estrogen levels can cause skin to begin to wrinkle. HRT is effective in maintaining smooth, youthful-looking skin, experts say.

The biggest concern for most women who are considering HRT is whether it will increase their risk for breast cancer. Various studies have come to different, often contradictory conclusions. But one study by researchers at the Centers for Disease Control and Prevention in Atlanta compiled the results of many other studies and came to the following conclusions: Current users may be at increased risk, but it appears that the risk is relative to how long a woman takes the hormones.

There does not appear to be an association with breast cancer in women who have taken it for less than 5 years, but women who have used it for over 15 years may have about a 30 percent increased risk. Women who used ERT in the past but are not currently taking it do not appear to be at increased risk for breast cancer.

What You Can Do

How do you decide? It's not easy, but here are some options to consider.

Find the right doctor. Doctors may vary in their approaches to HRT, so it's important to find one you're comfortable with and who respects your feelings and opinions, says Borton. Don't be afraid to shop around for a doctor and ask your friends about theirs.

Know your family history. In deciding about HRT, it's important to know your family history. Find out if anyone in your family has a history of heart disease, osteoporosis, breast cancer, or endometrial cancer. Tell your doctor.

Weigh your risks. Deciding on HRT is often a matter of balancing your risk for one disease against your risk for another. One solution is to try "to decide as a woman what you are at risk for and what your risk profile is and to make an intelligent decision about what diseases you ought to be preventing that you are likely to get," says David Felson, M.D., of the Boston University Arthritis Center.

Keep menstrual records. When women go on HRT, they often get their periods again, particularly if they are taking progesterone with estrogen. Hormone preparations can affect your flow, so record your bleeding pattern, says Brian Walsh, M.D., director of the Menopause Clinic at Brigham and Women's Hospital in Boston. Take a calendar, mark the days when you bleed, and show it to your doctor, so she can determine whether the timing and amount of flow are appropriate, he says.

Expect time for adjustment. It may take four to six weeks for the hormones to kick in and for you to feel an effect, says Dr. Walsh. And once you're on them, it may take several months to get your therapy adjusted so that your periods become regular.

Do those breast exams. All the questions about the connection between HRT and breast cancer aren't definitively answered. So cover your bases and perform monthly breast self-examinations; they'll enable you to detect breast cancer early if you develop it. Performing monthly breast self-examinations is one of the most important things a woman can do, says Dr. Walsh. "Most breast cancers are found by the woman herself, which is why it makes sense for her to examine her breasts once a month," he says. "That's 11 more times than her doctor has a chance to find a breast lump."

Get your mammograms. A mammogram is another way to detect breast cancer. Most doctors recommend that women have their first mammograms between the ages of 35 and 40. It's important for women on HRT to get mammograms on a regular basis, says Dr. Walsh. "People argue about how often and starting at what age, but by age 50, women should definitely be having mammograms at least every year." Mammograms "allow the breast cancer to be detected when it's small and potentially curable," he says.

Get a cancer check. Another type of follow-up test that women can have is called an endometrial biopsy. This checks the lining of the uterus, or endometrium, for cancer. Some doctors do a baseline biopsy at the start of HRT and then do a biopsy as an annual screening, although not all doctors do this with women who are receiving both estrogen and progesterone. The test is more important when a woman is taking just estrogen because the protective effect of progesterone is absent. Ask your doctor about her approach.

Get support. Other women going through menopause can be a tremendous source of support, says Borton. Talk to other women your age—either women you already know or those you meet in a support group—about their thinking, decisions, and experiences surrounding HRT, she says. Hearing other women's experiences can often help. Call a local hospital for information about support groups in your area or start one of your own.

HUMOR

It's No Joke—Laughter Is Healthy

Remember that game of Truth or Dare you played at Sally Winkler's sixth-grade party? You know, the one where Tommy Doyle had to kiss Sally's dog on the lips—and the dog kissed back? You laughed so hard that the little rubber bands on your braces popped out of your mouth.

At that tender age, you had already stumbled upon one of life's most potent natural age erasers: humor. In these hurry-up, way-too-serious days of adulthood, you can use a smile and a chuckle to help make yourself feel like a kid again. Humor can relax your body, ease your mind, relieve stress, and boost your creativity.

"A sense of humor is not a cure-all or end-all for healthy living," says Joel Goodman, Ed.D., director of the Humor Project in Saratoga Springs, New York. "But it's a great way to beat stress and worry, and it can really make you feel better about life. And the best part of all is that you can do it for yourself."

When something strikes you as funny, you laugh. And when you laugh, your body responds, says psychiatrist William F. Fry, M.D., associate clinical professor emeritus at Stanford University School of Medicine. You flex, then relax, 15 facial muscles plus dozens of others all over your body. Your pulse and respiration increase briefly, oxygenating your blood. And your brain experiences a decrease in pain perception, possibly associated with the production of painkilling, pleasure-giving endorphins.

There's evidence that laughter can spur your immune system, increasing the activity of lymphocytes and other "killer cells" (antibodies) and possibly raising levels of disease-fighting immunoglobulin A in your bloodstream, according to Kathleen Dillon, Ph.D., a psychologist and professor at Western New England College in Springfield, Massachusetts.

By the time you're done giggling, your body is calmer, your brain is clearer, and you may even discover that your headache or stiff neck has disappeared. Research shows that you also might be more capable of solving problems that seemed impossible a few grumpy minutes before. Not bad for a half-minute's work—if you can call laughing work.

The long-term effects of humor are harder to measure. The late author Norman Cousins credited laughter with helping him beat a potentially fatal connective tissue disease. After his diagnosis, Cousins moved into a hotel room, watched funny videos and movies, read funny books and magazines—and staged a stunning recovery.

Despite Cousins's success story, experts say that humor by itself won't cure disease or make you live longer. Still, many doctors have started working humor into treatments for everyone from cancer patients to people undergoing psychotherapy. "When used judiciously, I think it can indeed help with recovery," Dr. Fry says. "If nothing else, it makes the patient feel better for short periods of time."

Even if you're perfectly healthy, a well-honed sense of humor can raise your self-esteem—and maybe even make you more popular. "Humor can help you deal with unpleasant or difficult circumstances," Dr. Goodman says. "If you're able to laugh at yourself or a difficult situation, you're probably going to cope better and feel better in the long run."

Oh, and one other thing: Don't worry about developing laugh lines on your face. You're going to get some wrinkles no matter what you do, be it frowning or squinting or laughing. And specialists like Karen Burke, M.D., Ph.D., a dermatologist in private practice New York City, say "positive" wrinkles like laugh lines give your face some character—just as frown-faced people can develop creases that make them look perpetually glum.

Honing Your Funny Bone

Dear old Mrs. Stonyface. You remember her—the fourth-grade teacher whose idea of funny was spending a half-hour after school clapping erasers. Well, Dr. Goodman says that even she could have developed a working sense of humor.

"Everyone can laugh, though you might find that hard to believe," Dr. Goodman says. "The trick is to work on your sense of humor, to hone it, so that you can use it to your advantage."

So how do you make your life a little funnier? Experts offer these tips.

Focus on funny stuff. Try looking for humor in everyday life. It might help, Dr. Goodman says, to pretend you're Allen Funt of the old *Candid Camera* show for a few minutes each day. "Act like you're carrying around a video camera. Look for people who are doing funny things, or animals or children or anything that might make you laugh. The more you look for humor, the more you'll find it."

Take a child's-eye view. Buried under a pile of paperwork? If it looks high to you, think how towering—and wickedly cool—a seven-year-old would find it. Dr. Goodman says you should try picturing what most stressful adult situations would look like to a kid. The barking boss? The whining salesman? Your nagging Aunt Myrtle? They all look a little less threatening when seen with a childlike perspective.

Check your humor pulse. When it comes to laughter, it takes different jokes for different folks. Dr. Fry suggests spending a week or so to gauge your own sense of humor. Which comic strips make you laugh? Which movies? Which situations? Do you find yourself chuckling at your child's antics? Once you've figured it out, start a laugh library. Clip funny comics and stick them on your refrigerator door. Rent or buy funny movies or stand-up comedy routines. Shoot home videos of your wacko dog or your bumbling neighbor Bob.

"It's a simple thing to do," Dr. Fry says. "Still, many people don't think to add a little laughter to their lives, and that's really too bad because it really can make you feel better."

Meet your laugh quota. Dr. Goodman suggests trying to get 15 laughs a day, even if you have to look for the humor. "There's no magic in the number," he says. "It just seems about right to me. If you manage to reach your humor quota, you're probably feeling pretty good about life."

Even if you don't particularly feel like laughing, try it once in a while anyway. The reflexes, the smile, and the physiological changes your body will undergo just might make you feel better. You may even find yourself beginning to inject humor into tense situations—a great tool everywhere from the boardroom to the bedroom.

Choose wisely. Laughter can be contagious, but so can the plague. If you start making racist or ethnic jokes, people will start avoiding you. "Pick subjects that will bring people together in good humor," Dr. Fry says. "And never single someone out. That will make that person withdraw and could give him incentive to get back at you when you're most vulnerable."

Draw the line. Not everything is funny. And humor won't solve every dilemma. "There are times when you have to take things seriously," Dr. Goodman says. "Laughing at everything can be a form of avoidance. It helps to have a good attitude, sure, but there are certain times that we need to be sensible—like at funerals or in court or at important business meetings—and we need to consider if humor will work for or against us."

LEARNING

Have It Your Way

High school algebra? College chemistry? They're history. As an adult you can learn what you want, when you want, any way you want—and with a sense of fulfillment, accomplishment, and fun. And a feeling of youthfulness, too. Learning can bring back the feeling that the world is a boundless place, full of potential and hope.

Let's start by debunking one of the great myths of aging. Yes, you are losing 50,000 to 100,000 irreplaceable brain cells a day. But it doesn't make a bit of difference because you started with more than 100 billion. By the time you reach the age of 70, you'll still have 99 percent of your original total.

Experts say it's not the number of cells that counts, anyway. It's what you do with them. "The adage 'use it or lose it' applies to the mind as well as the muscles," says Marian Diamond, Ph.D., professor of neurosciences in the department of integrated biology at the University of California, Berkeley.

"Studies show that the area in the brain devoted to word understanding is significantly larger in the average college graduate than in the average high school graduate," Dr. Diamond says. "Why? Because college graduates spend more time working with words."

So there's no reason that adults can't learn as well as children do. In fact, being an adult often makes learning easier. "You can put things in context," says Ronald Gross, chairman of the University Seminar on Innovation in Education at Columbia University in New York City and author of *Peak Learning: A Master Course in Learning How to Learn.*

"When you're learning something, like philosophy, you have years of experience that will help you see where things fit in. You never had that edge when you were young," he says.

A Primer

The key to learning is overcoming the notion that the whole process is boring—or scary. "Learning can be life's greatest joy," Gross says. "It's what makes humans human. Why worry when you're doing it for yourself? Failing is not an issue. There's not going to be a test. Learn for the sake of learning, and you'll see how great you feel."

Ready to get started? Experts offer these tips.

Follow your heart. What have you always wanted to learn? Gardening? Spanish? Arc welding? Gross says you should make a list—and don't worry about whether the items seem important enough. Remember, you're learning for yourself. Pick one or two topics, save the rest for later, and take it from there.

Show some style. In school, everyone learned the same way: by being quiet, listening to the teacher, going home, and studying. Some people thrived and others didn't. That's because people learn in different ways. Do you like seminars with lots of people or one-on-one sessions? Are you sharpest at night or in the morning? Do you concentrate best with the radio playing softly in the background? "How you learn plays a large part in what you learn," Gross says. "Figure out your own style and make yourself comfortable."

Take your time. It's one thing to learn to play "Chopsticks" and another altogether to play Beethoven's Fifth Symphony. In other words, take your time. Otherwise, you may burn out on learning. "Too much stimulation loses its value," Dr. Diamond says. "By all means, enrich your mental life and keep your brain active, but allow yourself adequate time to assimilate new information."

Abandon ship. So you always wanted to learn to sail. And there you are, sailing solo, trimming the jib, and sheeting the main. But it's just not as much fun as you thought it would be. Head for the lifeboats and try something else. "There's no sense staying with something that isn't what you really want to do," Gross says.

But before you jump overboard, make sure it's for the right reason. Are you quitting because it's not interesting? Or are you having trouble with it because you're still learning the basics? Mastering a new task means sailing through some rough waters, but riding out the storm has its rewards.

Challenge yourself. Do you like only crossword puzzles that you can solve? Then you're not challenging yourself. While pushing too hard inhibits learning, not going hard enough can be stifling, too. Gross says you should always leave another bridge for yourself to cross. If you reach a goal, bask in the victory. Then set another goal and go after it.

Don't be afraid to ask. If you're taking a knitting class and don't know a knit from a purl, drop the needle and raise your hand. If you're not sure how hard to tighten an oil filter, call a garage and ask. Or consult the nearest librarian (a library card is one of the most powerful learning tools around). "Part of learning is knowing when to ask questions," Gross says. "Try to work things out for yourself. But you're not doing yourself any good if you reach a dead end and stay there."

LOW-FAT FOODS

Eating Lighter and Liking It

Most experts agree that a high-fat diet is a major cause of all kinds of killers, including cardiovascular disease, high blood pressure, diabetes, stroke, and some types of cancer. Fortunately, a wealth of scientific research shows that a low-fat diet reduces your risk of developing such chronic diseases. And a great number of studies also indicate that just a little less fat in your diet can lead to a trimmer, slimmer you. The bottom line: If health and longevity are among your goals, low-fat foods can help take you there.

So this all means that fat is a bad thing, right? Wrong! Actually, it's an essential nutrient that acts as a source of energy for the body and provides vital compounds to our body's cells so that they can carry out their daily functions. It's only when we eat too much fat that it has the potential to start trouble.

Most foods—even fruits and vegetables—contain some fat. It comes in three different forms: saturated, monounsaturated, and polyunsaturated. All three are equally fattening, but they have different health effects. Experts believe that we should eat fewer foods like butter that are high in saturated fats. "Saturated fats tend to raise the level of cholesterol in the blood, which raises the risk of heart disease," says Diane Grabowski-Nepa, R.D., a nutrition educator at the Pritikin Longevity Center in Santa Monica, California.

Monounsaturated fats—prevalent in canola and olive oils, avocados, and some nuts—do not seem to produce this rise in blood cholesterol levels, while studies have shown that polyunsaturated fats—

found in margarine, fish, and safflower and corn oils—can actually lower your cholesterol count. So if you're going to eat foods that contain fat, you're better off with those containing mostly monounsaturated or polyunsaturated fat.

Here are some foods Grabowski-Nepa recommends that you include on your low-fat menu.

POTATOES AND SWEET POTATOES. Baked spuds are a light and filling energy source. Just don't smother them with butter, sour cream, or gravy.

LEGUMES. Beans, peas, and lentils offer the same essential vitamins, minerals, and proteins found in meats but have virtually none of the fat.

FRUITS AND VEGETABLES. While there are a handful of high-fat fruits and vegetables (such as avocados and coconuts), most contain hardly any fat. And what little you find is usually monounsaturated or polyunsaturated.

WHOLE-GRAIN BREADS AND CEREALS, PASTAS, AND BROWN RICE. These foods are virtually fat-free, unless you overload them with butter and sauces. They are also your best sources of complex carbohydrates—the nutrients that give our bodies the most reliable and long-lasting form of energy—and fiber, which fights disease and aids digestion.

FISH AND FOWL. If you make fish, shellfish, and poultry your primary meat sources, you'll get all the protein and minerals of red meats but not nearly as much fat.

Lose the Fat, Keep the Flavor

Some simple, gradual changes to your eating habits are all it takes to make some major fat reductions. Here are some suggestions.

Don't add fat to a good thing. A lot of the foods we eat are naturally low in fat until we heap on those extras like butter, dressings, and creams. Start your fat-reducing program by using less of fatty condiments and other add-ons. "In a year's time, that'll make a big difference," says Susan Kayman, R.D., Dr.P.H., a dietitian and consultant with the Kaiser Permanente Medical Group in Oakland, California.

Season to perfection. Add herbs, spices, or tomato or lemon juice to liven up less flavorful foods without adding fat, says Grabowski-Nepa.

Choose low-fat cheese. Cheese is one of the most common fat boosters, says researcher Wayne Miller, Ph.D., director of the Indiana University Weight Loss Clinic in Bloomington. Most cheeses average about 66 percent of calories from fat, but some shoot well into the 80 percent range. You can generally distinguish high- and low-fat varieties by their color, Dr. Miller says; white cheeses like mozzarella, Swiss, ricotta, and Parmesan are lower in fat than yellow cheeses like Cheddar and American.

Minimize milk fat. Switching from whole milk to 1 percent can substantially cut your fat intake: 1 percent milk gets 23 percent of its calories from fat, while whole milk gets 48 percent. For better results, choose skim milk; it has virtually no fat. If you have trouble getting used to the taste of skim or low-fat milk, Dr. Miller suggests you make the transition slowly, combining it with regular whole milk and gradually increasing the amount of skim or 1 percent in the mixture.

Try low-fat versions of your favorites. "It's harder to totally swear off ice cream than to simply trade it for low-fat varieties or low-fat frozen yogurt," says Dr. Kayman. One study found that substituting fat-free products in just seven categories (cream cheese, sour cream, salad dressing, frozen desserts, processed cheese, baked sweets, and cottage cheese) cut fat intake by 14 percent a day.

Choose leaner meats. There's room for red meat in a low-fat diet if you make the right choices and eat it only two or three times a week. Best choices include cuts like London broil, eye of round steak, and sirloin tip, which get less than 40 percent of their calories from fat. Keep portions to about three or four ounces (the size of a deck of cards), trim all visible fat off before cooking, and prepare it by grilling, broiling, or baking.

Try not to fry. Cutting back on fried foods will cut a load of fat from your diet. Cooking anything in oil, even lean poultry, boosts its fat content considerably, says Dr. Miller. According to the U.S. Department of Agriculture, the average breaded fried chicken sandwich at a fast-food joint has 15 grams more fat than a quarter-pound burger. Go instead for broiled or baked foods, he suggests.

Skin the bird. Chicken and turkey are already leaner alternatives to beef and pork, says Grabowski-Nepa, but you make them even leaner if you peel the skin off before eating.

Fridge and skim. Grabowski-Nepa recommends an easy way to make gravies and broths less fatty: After cooking, just stick them in the refrigerator for several hours. Much of the fat will congeal and rise to the top, and all you'll have to do is skim it off.

Fill up when hunger strikes. If you replace fat with other filling, nutrient-dense foods, you can actually eat more and still maintain a healthy weight, says Annette Natow, R.D., Ph.D., of Nutrition Consultants in Valley Stream, New York, and co-author of *The Fat Attack*

Plan. Count on carbohydrates—pasta, cereals, breads, beans, and most fresh vegetables and fruits—to fill you up without the fat. Most of these foods in their whole or unprocessed forms are also full of fiber, which binds with fat and speeds it from your system.

Lose your sweet tooth. Many sugary foods are also high in fat. A chocolate bar, for example, gets most of its calories from fat, says Dr. Natow. Sweet cravings are often really fat cravings in disguise. If you want something sweet, try some fresh fruit or a bowl of sugared breakfast cereal with low-fat milk, she says. Or when you're cooking, use cocoa, which has less fat than baking chocolate.

MASSAGE

Much-Kneaded Relief

You've been waiting all week for this hour of ec-
stasy. Anxiety at work—rub, rub. Tension at home—stroke, stroke.
Those aching muscles and joints—tappity-tappity-tap. They're all
melting away with each pass of your massage therapist's hands.

After 45 minutes, that age-erasing magic has worked again. No
sore back. No stiff neck. You rise refreshed and relaxed, leaving behind
what feels like 20 years of pain and worries.

"Nothing makes you feel more rejuvenated than a massage," says
Madeline P. Rudy, a licensed massage therapist with Massage Therapy
in West Reading, Pennsylvania. "If you're looking for a way to put
yourself back in sync and feel younger, there isn't a better thing out
there."

Anyone will tell you that a massage feels great. Yet medical science
still doesn't know exactly why. "There's not a lot of research out there
yet," says Tiffany Field, Ph.D., director of the Touch Research Institute at the University of Miami School of Medicine. The institute is
the first organization in the country dedicated to studying massage's
medical benefits.

Dr. Field says that we have gained a few insights into the way massage works, however. For one thing, it seems to restrict the body's release of cortisol, a hormone that plays a big role in triggering stress reactions. The less cortisol you produce, the less stress you may feel, she
says. Massage also has been shown to improve the deep, resting phase
of sleep. And it may boost your production of serotonin, a hormone

linked to positive mood changes and improved immunity, Dr. Field says.

In a Touch Research Institute study of medical faculty and staff, 15 minutes of daily massage appeared to lessen anxiety, make people more alert, and increase the speed with which they could complete math problems. "The key to a better workforce," Dr. Field says, "could be regular massage."

The institute is working on a series of 34 studies, with hundreds of participants, that looks at massage therapy's effects on everything from depression and pregnancy to high blood pressure and migraine headaches. The studies also look at how massage therapy could help males who test positive for HIV (the virus that causes AIDS) improve their immune function.

For now, some doctors say that they need to know more about what massage can do before they start prescribing it as therapy.

"No one is willing to accept any nebulous explanation that involves the metaphors of energy, toxins, good vibes, or any other poetic verse," says Larry Dossey, M.D., co-chairman of the panel on Mind/Body Interventions, Office of Alternative Medicine at the National Institutes of Health in Bethesda, Maryland, and former chief of staff at Medical City Dallas Hospital in Dallas.

But that attitude may be changing. Many insurance companies now cover massage if a doctor orders it. And some massage therapists note that some of their best, most loyal clients are physicians.

Some Hands-On Advice

If you're thinking about trying massage therapy, Rudy says you should be prepared to spend anywhere from $25 to $65 per session, with a typical session lasting about 50 to 55 minutes. Go as often as you like or as often as you can afford. For more guidance, try these tips.

Shop carefully. The last place you want to end up in is a massage "parlor," with its creepy clientele and sometimes questionable practices. To find a reputable, qualified massage therapist, ask questions before you go. "Look in the phone book," Rudy says. "Make sure they're a member of the American Massage Therapy Association (AMTA). Ask if they went to accredited schools to learn massage. And always avoid places that offer 'discreet billing.' That's a sign that they may not be on the up-and-up."

The AMTA has a customer referral service that will help you find a registered massage therapist in your area. Write the group at 820 Davis Street, Suite 100, Evanston, IL 60201.

Pick your pleasure. When it comes to massage, there really are different strokes for different folks. Swedish massage—with its kneading, rubbing, and use of oils—is the method most people think of. But there's also shiatsu, or oriental massage, in which a therapist works pressure points along nerve pathways to relieve pain and stress (Rudy says some people may experience some discomfort with this method). There's specialized sports massage, which focuses on soothing overworked muscles and joints. And there's a grab bag of techniques and subtechniques like Rolfing, Feldenkrais, Trager, Alexander, and Aston-Patterning, which promote everything from body-lengthening to spine realignments to posture improvements.

"The key is to talk to therapists first," Rudy says. "You want to find someone whose specialty matches your needs. And you want to make sure they're legitimate."

Respect your limits. Massage is about relaxation. And let's face it: Some people just aren't comfortable disrobing for a Swedish massage. "Only go as far as what feels right," Rudy says. "Maybe you'll have to work your way up to it. This is your special time. Enjoy it."

Therapists should be conscious of your feelings. They should cover parts of the body they're not working on and should not touch your breasts or genital areas. They shouldn't ask you for intimate details of your life or give details of theirs. They're supposed to respect your wishes. If they don't, find another massage therapist.

"The whole thing," Rudy says, "is about health and well-being and feeling better. If there's tension or pressure in a relationship, go somewhere else."

Know when to say no. Massage isn't for everyone. AMTA guidelines say that people with phlebitis or other circulatory ailments, some forms of cancer or heart disease, infections, or fevers should not use massage therapy. In most cases, avoid massage for about three days after suffering a fracture or serious sprain. If you have any doubts, ask your physician.

MEDICAL CHECKUPS

Well Worth Your Time

Through regular checkups, you and your doctor can keep an eye out for developing problems and perhaps put a stop to them. Just as important, meeting with your doctor can give you a chance to discuss certain lifestyle factors that can make the difference between a long, vigorous life and a short one plagued with problems.

Getting a checkup seems simple enough, but where it can quickly start to resemble the quest for the Holy Grail is when you start looking for a doctor. What should you be looking for?

"Basically, anyone who holds himself out by training and practice as a primary care physician should be fully qualified to take care of checkups for normal, healthy adults," says Douglas Kamerow, M.D., director of the Clinical Preventive Services Staff for the Office of Disease Prevention and Health Promotion in the U.S. Public Health Service. "But in my opinion, there are really only two groups that are qualified by their training to do so—general internists and family physicians."

For women, some experts would narrow the list even further. "My number one choice would be a general internist," says Lila Wallis, M.D., clinical professor of medicine at Cornell University Medical College, former president of the American Medical Women's Association, and founder of the National Council of Women's Health in New York City. "And not just any general internist, but one who has had special training in office gynecology and the psychological needs of female patients."

Interestingly, a gynecologist might not be a woman's best choice. "While general internists and family practitioners already have a firm knowledge of the rest of the body, gynecologists specialize specifically in women's sexual organs and reproductive tract," notes Dr. Wallis. "This gives them far more to learn than the other two to become a primary care physician."

What Your Doctor Needs to Know

Sherlock Holmes may have been able to get to the truth based on the merest of clues, but your doctor needs solid information. You can best provide that information by doing a bit of homework before your visit.

Keep a food log. When it comes to health habits, the murkiest information tends to surround diet. "If you know you're going in for a checkup and plan on discussing diet, it's not a bad idea to keep a precise food log for a week beforehand," suggests Dr. Kamerow. "Don't change your eating habits, just keep track of them. It's the little forgettable things like snacks that add up to a lot of dietary fat, and it's these things that you'll need to focus on when talking to your doctor."

Climb your family tree. "People with a family history of certain health problems may be at greater risk of developing them, and it's reasonable to screen these people more regularly or earlier for these diseases," says Dr. Kamerow.

While there may well be hundreds of diseases that can be passed along genetically, there are only a few that you generally need to be concerned with. "For women, breast cancer is a primary concern," says Dr. Kamerow. "The U.S. Preventive Services Task Force does not recommend mammograms before the age of 50. But doctors may want to make an exception for women who are at high risk by evidence that their mother or sister had it, especially if the cancer was premenopausal."

Osteoporosis is another concern for women. "A family history of osteoporosis might predispose me to suggest a bone mineral density study at menopause, which I might not normally use routinely," says Dr. Wallis.

For men, "studies at Johns Hopkins University have shown that a man whose father has had prostate cancer is at 2½ times the risk for developing the disease himself," says Kenneth Goldberg, M.D., founder and director of the Male Health Center in Dallas and author of *How Men Can Live as Long as Women: Seven Steps to a Longer and Better Life.*

"And if both his father and grandfather had it, the risk jumps to 9 times."

Testicular cancer is another hereditary pitfall for men. "Research in Great Britain has shown that men whose fathers have had cancer of the testicles are at four times the risk of developing it themselves," notes Dr. Goldberg. "And the genetic tie appears even stronger between brothers."

The final condition for both sexes to really watch for is heart disease. Among men, especially, "if you have a father or grandfather who had a heart attack in his forties, that would be good to know about because you might want to spend more time talking to your doctor about your cholesterol and other factors that might elevate your risk," suggests Dr. Kamerow.

Prepare your files. You'll want to make sure your doctor has records from any other physicians you may have visited. You'll also want to inform him of any medications that you are taking and any problems that you feel you may be experiencing because of them. You may also want to prepare a list of current health complaints, complete with symptoms and dates, if possible.

Getting the Most from It

"For women, one of the most important components of the physical is a breast examination," says JoAnn E. Manson, M.D., associate professor of medicine at Harvard Medical School and co-director of women's health at Brigham and Women's Hospital, both in Boston. "And, of course, a pelvic exam and Pap smear."

It's important for men have the abdomen and groin checked for a hernia, says Dr. Goldberg. The physician should also examine a man's testicles and penis for cancer or other abnormalities, including warts or sores.

For both sexes, experts recommend that the examination include the following procedures.

- Measurement of blood pressure, weight, and height

- Inspection of the tongue and gums for any signs of oral cancer or need for dental care

- A check of the neck artery for pulse and for bruits (abnormal sounds that can indicate a clogged artery)

- Inspection of the neck area for thyroid size and nodules that might indicate possible cancer

- Examination of the skin, especially in sun-exposed areas, for any signs of skin cancer

- Stethoscope examination of the chest for heart sounds and lung congestion, crackles, or wheezes

"In some people, especially those who are young and healthy, it may be less important to check the liver, kidneys, spleen, and reflexes and test for signs of nerve damage," says Dr. Manson. "The need for many of these tests depends on age, prior medical history, and risk factors."

When it comes to the more exotic blood and urine tests, electrocardiograms, and x-rays, the U.S. Preventive Services Task Force (of which Dr. Kamerow is staff director) does not routinely recommend them for healthy patients.

The only place that there is some hubbub is in the area of rectal examinations and prostate specific antigen (PSA) tests. "We don't recommend rectal examination," says Dr. Kamerow, "but some groups feel that starting at age 40, this should be a routine part of the checkup."

Dr. Goldberg is part of the "pro" group. "Beginning at age 40, every man should have a digital rectal exam every year. It's the first line in detecting prostate cancer, which is the second leading cancer in men." Dr. Goldberg also recommends screening for PSA at age 50. "It's produced exclusively by the prostate gland, so it's a sensitive marker for prostate cancer and other prostate problems," he says. "After age 50, your blood should be analyzed for PSA once a year. And if you've got hereditary risk factors, you should start at 40."

As women reach menopause, one test might be added to their routine checkup. "There is no better way of determining how a woman's bones will fare later than a bone mineral density study at menopause," says Dr. Wallis. "If the patient exhibits any risk factors such as a family history of osteoporosis, a pale complexion, red or blonde hair, northern European origin, lack of exposure to sun, lack of exercise, or a lack of calcium intake, I would definitely suggest she undergo it."

A bone mineral density study takes anywhere from five minutes to a half-hour (depending on the technology used) and is a painless, noninvasive scan performed by machines that use low-dose radiation to measure bone mass.

The other change in a woman's checkup routine happens at 40. At that age, most doctors recommend regular mammograms. "Some would also recommend a fecal occult blood test and a sigmoidoscopy to screen for colorectal cancer," says Dr. Kamerow.

Taking the Doctor's Advice Home

"Outside of the few tests and shots that you should get, the most important thing that can be done at a checkup is to team up with your doctor and take stock of your health habits," states Dr. Kamerow. The big four topics of discussion should be exercise, diet, sexual practices, and vices such as smoking and drinking, he says.

If you smoke, talk to your doctor about ways to quit. The same goes for "recreational" drugs, excessive use of medications such as sedatives and diet pills, and alcohol abuse. If you are prone to adventurous sex, have a sobering conversation about safe sex. Diet? Haul out that food diary and go over it in detail. As for exercise, ask your doctor for tips on how to incorporate more physical activity into your life.

If you think that all of this is taking up too much of your doctor's valuable time, forget it. "The most important thing that goes on at a checkup is the counseling and the activity that the patient then does because of that counseling," says Dr. Kamerow. "Doctors are beginning to realize that the most healing thing they can do is provide information and motivation."

OPTIMISM

A Proven Power for Health

Optimism is not about ignoring what's real but about becoming aware of your thoughts about why things happen, says Martin Seligman, Ph.D., professor of psychology and director of clinical training at the University of Pennsylvania in Philadelphia and author of *Learned Optimism.*

What's really at the heart of optimism, Dr. Seligman says, is how you explain negative experiences to yourself. When something bad happens to a pessimist, he's likely to get into a sort of dark and hopeless mental muttering that has him thinking things like "It's all my fault, it's permanent, and everything is ruined." The optimist's explanation? "It was bad luck, it will pass, and I'll handle it differently next time."

Optimism can give you real resilience as you get older. "Research has shown that optimistic attitudes and beliefs are associated with fewer illnesses and quicker recovery from illness," says Christopher Peterson, Ph.D., professor of psychology at the University of Michigan in Ann Arbor and author of *Health and Optimism.* Pessimism, however, may lower your resistance to illness, increase your chances of heart disease, and even shorten your life, researchers say.

There's a lot to be said for cultivating optimistic attitudes now, before the challenges of old age arrive. Some researchers speculate that pessimism begins to have a negative effect on health in middle age, around ages 35 to 50.

Learning How to Hope

If grubbing in the garden of gloom has been your lifelong habit, here's how to cultivate a more upbeat attitude, say the experts.

Notice how your friends feel. Look at their attitudes, says Dr. Peterson. "Optimism and pessimism are both contagious states. So to 'catch' optimism, associate as much as possible with positive people."

Negotiate with negative types. You can't be the only optimist in a family of pessimists, Dr. Peterson says. You're likely to cave in and become a pessimist yourself. So if it's a family member who spouts negativity all day long, try saying, "It really drives me crazy when you talk like this. Can we be negative once a week instead?"

Savor your successes. We're trained to be modest, says Dr. Peterson, but there's no need to belittle your own triumphs. Instead, you can say to yourself, "I worked really hard, I did a good job, and I'm proud of myself." That's the optimistic way of thinking about good events that you brought about by your own efforts.

Face facts, but never give up. Optimism doesn't mean that you're not in touch with hard facts, says William Rakowski, Ph.D., a gerontologist at the Center for Gerontology and Health Care Research at Brown University in Providence, Rhode Island. "Be realistic about what's happened in your life: 'I was a victim of circumstance there,' 'That was my fault,' 'That wasn't.'" And then use optimism to resolve that, in spite of it all. Tell yourself, 'With effort, initiative, and good luck, I will still have good things to look forward to,'" he says.

Make the best of hard times. Some people face a great deal of adversity and still call themselves optimists, Dr. Rakowski says. Why? "When you're optimistic, you're also believing 'I can make the most of what I've got,'" he says. "Sometimes you need to redefine your objectives and let go of an initial expectation. Then your basic objective is still to make the most of what you have."

Distance yourself from your beliefs. It is essential to realize that your beliefs are just that—beliefs, not facts, Dr. Seligman says. If a jealous rival at work said to you, "You're a terrible manager and you'll never make it in this business," you'd know to ignore his insults. But what about the spiteful things we say to ourselves? They can be just as baseless as jealous insults, only it's bad thinking—a mental reflex that you don't have to find convincing. "Check out the accuracy of your reflexive beliefs and argue with yourself," he says.

Learn your optimism A-B-C. Three things happen when you face a tough situation, and A-B-C is a good way to remember the pattern, says Dr. Seligman. You respond to *a*dversity with a *b*elief, which determines the *c*onsequence. For example, you're on the phone trying to make a sale, and your first caller hangs up on you—adversity. When you respond with an optimistic belief, such as "Oh well, that's one no out of the way; it brings me closer to the yes," then the likely consequence is that you'll feel relaxed and energetic. Compare that with a knee-jerk negative belief, such as "I'll never get any better at this," which produces an equally negative consequence (you feel lousy about yourself).

Derail negative thoughts. When a persistent negative thought runs repeatedly through your mind, try techniques like these: Smack your palm hard on your desk and say—loudly—"Stop!" Or put a rubber band around your wrist and snap it every time you have the thought. Or write down the thought and set aside a time to think it over later. These techniques can stop a bout of pessimism before it starts.

Give a little. If painful circumstances have made you unhappy, doing what you can to help others may give you a more optimistic view, says Dr. Rakowski. Whether you do volunteer work or simply offer to listen to a friend's troubles, there's a real sense of fulfillment in giving that can lift you out of your pain, he says.

Get help for depression. "If you're a real pessimist, odds are you're fairly depressed," says Dr. Peterson. "Undergoing therapy for depression can make you healthier and improve your life." Cognitive behavioral therapy, during which you learn to challenge defeatist ways of thinking, is particularly helpful in turning depression around, he says. Chronically unhappy people do a running negative commentary on their lives that they're often not aware of. A therapist can teach you ways to divert yourself when you get in these moods. These techniques won't reduce the frequency of episodes of depression you have but will shorten them, he says. And in some cases, a prescription for antidepressant medication may help.

RELAXATION

Mother Nature's Secret Life-Enhancer

Taking a few minutes each day to relax and let life's strains roll off isn't a luxury; it's a necessity if you want to stay vigorous, productive, and healthy.

"There are three main things you can do to prolong your life. One is to exercise, one is to maintain proper nutrition, and the other is to relax. Relaxation can definitely help you age better. It's important for preventing a wide variety of disorders and for increasing your effectiveness and efficiency in life," says Frank J. McGuigan, Ph.D., director of the Institute for Stress Management at United States International University in San Diego. "I don't think there's any question that relaxation can have a positive effect on phobias, depression, anxiety, high blood pressure, ulcers, colitis, headaches, and lower back pain."

How to Chill Out

Here are a few basic strategies to help you get some relaxation into your life.

Snuff the smokes. "Our studies show that smoking causes blood vessels to clamp down and restrict blood flow," says Robert S. Eliot, M.D., director of the Institute of Stress Medicine in Jackson Hole, Wyoming, and author of *From Stress to Strength: How* *to Lighten Your Load and Save Your Life.* "If there's a single thing that people can do to feel less stressed and more relaxed, it's kicking the habit."

Whittle your weight. "It's hard to feel relaxed if you're carrying around extra weight," Dr. Eliot says. "Your clothes don't feel comfortable and your body image suffers." Being overweight also contributes to high blood pressure, heart disease, and diabetes.

Team up with carbos. "Protein seems to raise energy levels and keep you alert," Dr. Eliot says. "So if you have a hamburger late at night, you'll probably be rehashing yesterday's sales meeting until dawn." Carbohydrates, on the other hand, trigger the release of hormones that will relax you. So if you want to unwind at night, eat a plate of spaghetti, baked beans, or other complex carbohydrates for dinner.

Write it down. Over a dozen studies have shown that if you write about your problems, you can help relieve stress, improve your immunity, make fewer visits to the doctor, and have a more optimistic view of life, says James Pennebaker, Ph.D., professor of psychology at Southern Methodist University in Dallas. Spend 20 minutes a day writing how you feel about things that are really upsetting you. Then when you're finished, throw the paper away. You may feel a sense of relief when you're done.

Time is on your side. "Every time you look at a clock or your watch during a day, take a deep breath while consciously raising and lowering your shoulders or dropping your jaw," says Saki Santorelli, Ed.D., associate director of the Stress Reduction Clinic at the University of Massachusetts Medical Center in Worcester. "That probably takes 10 seconds and will serve as a reminder to you that you can be at ease while going about your daily schedule."

Laugh it off. Humor is a powerful relaxation technique, Dr. Eliot says. Laughter triggers the release of endorphins, chemicals in the brain that produce feelings of euphoria. It also suppresses the production of cortisol, a hormone released when you're under stress that indirectly raises blood pressure. So share a good laugh with a friend or keep a handy file of humorous anecdotes and drawings in a drawer that you can quickly pull out.

Snooze away. Get plenty of uninterrupted sleep, Dr. Eliot advises. If you get less sleep than you need, you might wake feeling tense and incapable of coping with life's basic hassles. Try to get at least six to eight hours of sleep each night. But avoid alcohol or sleeping pills. They can interfere with your natural sleeping patterns and actually cause you to have a less restful night.

Going with the Flow

There are many methods available for the development of calmness and stability. No single method is right for everyone. The key is finding one that feels comfortable to you. "I feel that it is important to set aside a block of time each day to practice these methods and then incorporate them into your daily life. Often, these can be so unobtrusive that most people won't know that you're doing anything special," says Dr. Santorelli. Here are some ideas.

Pay attention to your breath. This simple form of meditation can be very calming, Dr. Santorelli says. Sit in a comfortable chair or on the floor so that your back, neck, and head are straight but not rigid. Exhaling deeply, allow the inhalation to come naturally. Simply pay attention to the gentle rising and falling of your abdomen, the movement of your ribs, or the sensation of the breath moving through your nostrils. Focus your mind on your breathing. If your mind starts to wander, gently escort your mind back to your breathing.

Climb every mountain. Visualization and imagery can encourage the development of calmness and well-being, Dr. Santorelli says. Closing your eyes, once again become aware of your breath and bring to mind a favorite mountain in your life. It could be one you've climbed or yearned to visit. Allow your body to become the stable foundation, sloping sides, and summit. Feel yourself steady, solid, grounded. As your sense of stability and steadiness grows, allow the weather to vary. Although the weather changes, notice that the mountain remains steady and dignified. "This image helps you realize that you can feel stable and secure and endure any storm that life has in store for you," Dr. Santorelli says.

Move that body. Exercise triggers the release of endorphins, but exercising the mind and body simultaneously may produce even better results, according to researchers at the University of Massachusetts Medical Center in Worcester. They asked 40 sedentary people to begin walking 35 to 40 minutes a day, three times a week, while listening to relaxation tapes. The tapes guided the walkers through a meditation that helped them focus on the one-two rhythm of their steps. The researchers concluded that this routine provoked more feelings of euphoria and reduced anxiety than in a matched group who exercised at the same intensity but didn't listen to the tapes.

Focusing your mind on a repetitive rhythm like exercise gives the brain a chance to restore itself and calm down. To try it, pick an exercise (such as walking, running, swimming, or climbing stairs) that has a natural rhythm. Focus your attention on that rhythm—even to the point of repeating the words "one, two" in your head in cadence with the exercise. Try to stay in that rhythm. As with breathing or other types of meditation, your mind may start to wander after a couple of minutes. If it does, refocus your attention on the repetitive movement of the exercise, says Herbert Benson, M.D., associate professor of medicine at Harvard Medical School, chief of the behavioral medicine division at Beth Israel Deaconess Medical Center, both in Boston, and author of *The Relaxation Response*. Try doing this 20 minutes a day, three times a week.

Unleash those muscles. There are about 1,030 skeletal muscles in the body. When you feel under stress, these muscles naturally contract and create tension. One way to counteract that is with progressive relaxation. By systematically flexing and releasing muscles, progressive relaxation can whisk that tension right out of your body.

Although there are many variations, Martha Davis, Ph.D., a psychologist at Kaiser Permanente Medical Center in Santa Clara, California, and co-author of *The Relaxation and Stress Reduction Workbook*, suggests this approach: Clench your right fist as tightly as you can. Keep it clenched for about 10 seconds, then release. Feel the looseness in your right hand and notice how much more relaxed it feels than when you tensed it. Do the same thing with your left hand, then clench both fists at the same time. Bend your elbows and tense your arms. Release and let your arms hang at your sides. Continue this process by tensing then relaxing your shoulders and neck and wrinkling then relaxing your forehead and brows. Then squeeze your eyes and clench your jaw before moving on to tense then relax your stomach, lower back, thighs, buttocks, calves, and feet. It should take about 10 minutes to complete the entire sequence. Try to do these exercises twice a day.

Stretch them, too. Unlike progressive relaxation, which contracts muscles, gentle stretching allows muscles to stretch and relax. That's better for some people, particularly those with chronic muscle pain, says Charles Carlson, Ph.D., professor of psychology at the University of Kentucky in Lexington.

"If you tense a muscle that is already in pain, you'll likely just create more pain. That doesn't help you relax," Dr. Carlson says. "Gentle stretching does two things. First, if you gently stretch a muscle and release it, it will generally relax. But secondly, when you focus your attention on doing the stretch, it also helps the mind relax. Muscle stretching should always be done slowly and without pain. There should be no overstretching or bouncing of muscles."

RELIGION
AND SPIRITUALITY

The Strength of an Ageless Soul

Whether you head for a familiar pew or take a nontraditional path, having a spiritual life can provide a powerful force for health. Faith can help fend off many forms of physical illness as well as take the emotional edge off aging, experts say.

You don't have to belong to an organized religion to benefit from a spiritual life. Private and public expressions of spirituality—from meditation and prayer to attending religious services—increase emotional fulfillment while helping to relieve stress and depression. They also decrease your risk of heart disease and cancer.

What matters most in gaining these benefits is to experience your own spirituality in your own way, says Mark Gerzon, author of *Coming into Our Own: Understanding the Adult Metamorphosis.* Perhaps your sense of the sacred has more to do with nature walks or loving relationships than participating publicly in religious rites.

One way of searching for a sense of wholeness is through meditation or prayer, both of which have been shown to decrease heart rate and blood pressure and to help you cope better with stress. Health experts have known for years that stress contributes to many physical problems including nausea, diarrhea, constipation, high blood pressure, and heart rhythm abnormalities. Studies have shown that strong religious beliefs go a long way to relieve stress—even if you simply hold your beliefs privately. But the stress-relieving effects of faith are most powerful, experts say, when you are regularly involved with a religious community.

Researchers at Ben Gurion University of the Negev and Soroka Medical Center in Beersheba, Israel, studied how 230 members of a religious kibbutz community coped with stressful life events. People within the community found that their individual faith and coping skills were strengthened by the support the community offered. And that resulted in quicker recovery from stress—including the stresses associated with getting older.

Spirituality offers particularly strong protection against a major killer—heart disease, says Dave Larson, M.D., adjunct associate professor of psychiatry at Duke University Medical Center in Durham, North Carolina.

A study of 85 women and 454 men in Jerusalem found that people who define themselves as "secular" (nonreligious) have a greater risk of heart disease than those who follow the path of Orthodox Judaism. Even after the researchers accounted for smoking habits and cholesterol and blood pressure levels, a strong association between lowered heart disease risk and religious practice remained for both sexes.

Although the researchers are unsure which aspects of belief are responsible, they speculate that the strong social support system of traditional Orthodox communities, like those of many other types of congregations, plays a heart-protecting role, probably by reducing isolation and stress.

An active spiritual or religious life also helps shield you from mental and emotional illness. Dr. Larson and his research team reviewed more than 200 studies on religious commitment and mental health. Their research revealed that people who are religious have lower rates of depression, alcoholism, suicide, and drug use than less religious people do.

How to Embrace the Spirit

You may feel a growing yearning for a deeper sense of meaning in your life. Here's how to rekindle your spiritual flame.

Begin at the beginning. Before you recommit to your childhood religion or embrace another faith, examine it, says Alan Berger, Ph.D., director of Jewish studies in the department of religion at Syracuse

University in New York. "Ask yourself, 'What is it that my tradition teaches?'" he says. "Don't feel you have to accept it, but do know it." **Go beyond the "don'ts."** If religion seems like a series of rules or thou-shalt-nots, Dr. Berger says, "You need to unskew your view. Go find yourself a better teacher, a new community. Read the texts yourself or with a partner and uncover the various levels of meaning. Understand that life is a fluid and dynamic experience that people need help with. Religion is the attempt to search for meaning in an otherwise chaotic universe."

Accept yourself. "It's fine to say, 'I don't really know what I am spiritually,'" says Brother Guerric Plante, a monk at the Abbey of Gethsemane in New Haven, Kentucky. "Honesty has everything to do with spiritual growth." Once you're open with yourself about any confusion you feel, the way will become more clear.

Search with others. Read the religion and support group announcements in your newspaper to find a group or organization that may offer help for your spiritual search, Brother Plante says. "Faith can come through others—their example, their talk, their interest in others. Group therapy, religious services, or even a 12-step group for addiction can rekindle a spiritual life if you're sincerely searching."

Meditate or pray. Clear time from your schedule to sit in quiet contemplation and listen to the stillness within you, says Gerzon. "If we derive meaning and purpose in life only from doing, we're in trouble," he says. "We need to find it from being, and meditation is a good way to start learning about how to simply be."

Broaden your view. Sometimes just encouraging your sense of curiosity and wondering about life will lead you to spiritual truths. When you ponder some of the age-old questions such as "Why am I here?" or "What is the meaning of life?" you encourage your spiritual insight to unfold, says Gerzon.

Go against your grain. You're more likely to grow spiritually if you seek out activities that are different from what you usually do all day, says John Buehrens, a minister for more than 20 years and president of the Unitarian Universalist Association in Beacon, Massachusetts. If you spend your day locked away from others in a corporate office, then serving a meal to the needy might be just what you need. But if you're a lawyer at a free clinic or a social worker, you may benefit more from a religious discussion group, he says.

Buehrens's own spiritual discipline? "I'm a pointy-headed, pear-shaped intellectual," he says. "So one of my spiritual disciplines is getting some regular exercise. It really is a time of meditation and prayer for me."

Care about others. You need to get out of yourself to feel spiritually healthy, Buehrens says. "That's why community is so important to real spiritual growth because we're drawn out of ourselves. We'll never find peace along religious, racial, and ethnic lines unless we do this." His advice for isolated seekers? "Go help in a soup kitchen, go visit a nursing home, and get your nose out of your navel," he says.

Keep a spiritual journal. Writing in a daily journal about your spiritual questions, doubts, beliefs, and experiences can illuminate the meaning and value in your life, says Buehrens. "You may find that your subconscious is trying to get through to you with more life-enhancing and creatively responsible methods."

Don't be afraid to question. "All spiritual traditions try to teach an enhanced awareness of being, greater spiritual vitality, and deeper compassion for other people," Buehrens says. But any spiritual community that doesn't respect questioning or the importance of your individual conscience may be an unhealthy one, he says. His advice? Follow your own conscience to the spiritual path that's right for you.

RESISTANCE TRAINING

Give Your Life a Lift

Resistance training, otherwise known as weight lifting, improves muscle strength and endurance, qualities that will enable you to do the activities you love well into old age. It can also help improve your cholesterol level, enhance your bone strength, maintain or decrease weight, and improve your body image and self-esteem.

"If people stay with it, continue to be active, and continue to do activities that stress the muscles, they can fight off some of the effects of aging," says Alan Mikesky, Ph.D., an exercise physiologist and professor at Indiana University School of Physical Education in Indianapolis. "People can continue to do things they enjoy in life longer—and maintain their performance in what they're doing."

One of the major—and most obvious—benefits of resistance training is its effect on muscle strength. Maintaining or increasing muscle strength is crucial to maintaining independence as we age, says Miriam Nelson, Ph.D., a research scientist and exercise physiologist at the Jean Mayer USDA Human Nutrition Research Center on Aging at Tufts University in Boston. Adequate muscle strength is what enables you to do things like carry your own luggage, climb stairs, and get in and out of bed.

Resistance training increases muscle strength by putting more strain on a muscle than it's used to. This increased load stimulates the growth of small proteins inside each muscle cell that play a central role in the ability to generate force. "When you lift weights, you stress or challenge the muscle cells, and they adapt by making more force-generating proteins," says Dr. Mikesky.

Weight training also helps improve muscle endurance, says Dr. Mikesky, so in addition to giving you the strength you need to lift a suitcase, it will give you the endurance you need to carry that suitcase for a longer period of time.

It doesn't take long to improve muscle strength, says Dr. Mikesky. "You can increase strength very quickly, in as little as 2 to 3 weeks." Noticeable increases in muscle size take longer—about 6 to 8 weeks. Some studies have shown strength increases of 100 percent or more in 12 weeks, he says. The bad news is that you can lose strength gains just as quickly. "If you miss a week of workouts and go back and put the same weight on, it's harder," he says.

There are different theories on the best type of resistance training program to follow. A lot of it depends on your individual goals. In general, lifting a heavy weight in three sets of 8 to 12 repetitions is the best way to build strength. And lifting a lighter weight for more repetitions helps to build endurance and tone.

Weight training can also give your cardiovascular health a lift, experts say. Studies on the effect of weight training on cholesterol profiles are controversial, says Dr. Mikesky, but some studies suggest an improvement in cholesterol levels that's similar to that of endurance training, he says.

While researchers don't fully understand how weight training lowers cholesterol, one means might be its effect on body composition and weight, says Janet Walberg-Rankin, Ph.D., associate professor in the exercise science program in the division of health and physical education at Virginia Polytechnic Institute and State University in Blacksburg. Weight training sometimes leads to weight loss and the reduction of body fat, and that can cause cholesterol to drop, she says.

Resistance training can certainly have an effect on your body composition. Muscles burn more calories than fat, so by increasing muscle mass, you increase your metabolic rate and can burn calories and reduce fat tissue.

Resistance training puts stress on bone as well as muscle and thereby helps increase bone mineral mass and prevent osteoporosis, experts say. While aerobic weight-bearing exercise like walking and running helps maintain bone strength in the legs and hips, it's less effective on the spine and upper body. Resistance training helps maintain bone strength in those areas, says Dr. Walberg-Rankin.

Weight training may be a very effective way to boost self-esteem because feedback is immediate. In addition to being able to see muscle growth and improved muscle tone, progress is easy to detect. "You know in two weeks when you can lift more weights on a machine," says Dr. Walberg-Rankin. That's a little easier to detect than an improvement in your aerobic fitness, she says.

How to Get to It

Why wait when you can be lifting weights? Here are some tips for getting started.

Check it out. Your physical health, that is. If you're going to start a resistance-training program, see your doctor for a physical first, says Dr. Walberg-Rankin. Your doctor will do a physical exam and take a health history. If you have a history of osteoporosis, heart disease, or high blood pressure, be sure to mention it.

Don't go it alone. If you're going to start resistance training, you must get instruction from an experienced person, says Dr. Walberg-Rankin. If you belong to a health club, get a qualified instructor to help you. Look for certification from the American College of Sports Medicine or the National Strength and Conditioning Association. The instructor can help you decide on the best resistance training method for you and get you started on a program. If you are doing a home program with a gym machine or dumbbell weights, consult a video on proper weight-lifting techniques, she says. If you're interested in using resistance tubing (elastic bands), consult a physical therapist or exercise physiologist.

Be sure to breathe. While you're lifting, do not hold your breath, says Dr. Walberg-Rankin. Breathe in or out while lifting, she says. It doesn't really matter when you inhale or exhale, she says, just be sure to do it throughout the exercise. Holding your breath can cause your blood pressure to skyrocket, which can be very dangerous.

Start out light. "Start low and progress slowly," says Dr. Mikesky. That means start with a lighter weight that you can lift 10 to 15 times and then progress slowly over the weeks to lifting heavier weights.

Keep at it. If you're persistent and consistent about lifting, your strength should gradually increase over a number of months. You may reach a point where you plateau, says physical therapist Mark Taranta, director of the Physical Therapy Practice in Philadelphia. But it's important to keep lifting even at that plateau level to maintain strength.

Do lifts you like. There are many different exercises for each muscle group. "If you don't like an exercise, don't stay with it. Find one you like," says Dr. Mikesky.

Lower slowly. Focus on lowering the weight slowly. That half of the movement, called a negative (or eccentric) contraction, actually stimulates more muscle growth, says Dr. Nelson. One method is to take a longer time lowering the weight than raising it. Try lifting the weight to the count of three and lowering it to the count of four.

Get started. It's never too late to start weight training, says Dr. Mikesky. Muscle can adapt and increase in strength well into your older years, he says. Research at Tufts University has shown strength gains between 100 and 200 percent in individuals well into their nineties.

SEX

It Does a Body Good

It doesn't take a genius to figure out that the bliss you feel after sex is good for you. Scientists believe sex is a great tension reliever because it releases chemicals in the brain called endorphins. Endorphins are natural painkillers that calm you, create a sense of euphoria, and temporarily melt down your stress, says Helen S. Kaplan, M.D., Ph.D., director of the Human Sexuality Teaching Program at New York Hospital–Cornell Medical Center in New York City.

Medical researchers also say that regular sex can soothe chronic aches and pains, spur creativity, rev up energy, and make you feel youthful. "Anything that makes you feel good, alive, and physically excited will make you feel more youthful," says Lonnie Barbach, Ph.D., a sex therapist and psychologist in private practice in San Francisco and writer of the video *Sex after Fifty*.

Making Great Sex Better

For good sex, keep your body healthy by avoiding smoking and fatty foods, which can clog blood vessels and make arousal and orgasm difficult. Here are some other tips to add zing to your sex life.

Get physical. Aerobic exercise three times a week, for 20 to 30 minutes a session, can improve your sex drive and performance, says Roger Crenshaw, M.D., a psychiatrist and sex therapist in private practice in La Jolla, California.

Talk it over. Communicate with your partner about what you want sexually, then listen while your mate does the same. If you don't say what you really want, then don't expect your partner to please you, says Shirley Zussman, Ed.D., a sex and marital therapist and co-director of the Association for Male Sexual Dysfunction in New York City. Keep it positive: "I enjoy sex with you, but I have some ideas about making it even better." And don't hesitate to *show* your partner what you want.

Broaden your horizons. "Intercourse is overemphasized as a sexual activity," says Marty Klein, Ph.D., a licensed marriage counselor and sex therapist in Palo Alto, California, and author of *Ask Me Anything: A Sex Therapist Answers the Most Important Questions of the '90s.* So take time to kiss, hug, caress, hold hands, talk, or do other sexually pleasing activities.

Make time for whoopee. Some couples say they just don't have time for sex. Rather than letting sex get lost in the daily grind, schedule time for it, says Michael Seiler, Ph.D., assistant director of the Phoenix Institute in Chicago and co-author of *Inhibited Sexual Desire.*

Check your hang-ups at the door. "Leave work, religion, and your performance expectations outside the bedroom door," Dr. Barbach suggests. "Simply go into the bedroom with your body and your feelings. Focus on the emotional connection you have with your partner and the pleasure your body has in store."

Just do it. "Most men would benefit from not worrying whether they're doing it right," Dr. Klein says. "You'll have better sex if you simply focus on your own body and do what feels good."

Keep it fun. "The Eskimos call sex laughing time," Dr. Zussman says. "Sex can be fun, frivolous, and relaxing." Concentrate on having a good time with your partner, and sex will be much more like laughing time than working overtime.

Put the squeeze on orgasms. Kegel exercises can help men sustain their erections and control orgasms, says Cynthia Mervis Watson, M.D., a clinical instructor in the department of family medicine at the University of Southern California in Los Angeles and author of *Love Potions.* Kegels strengthen the pubococcygeus muscles around the genital area. These are muscles that run from the pubic bone along the scrotum and back to the anus. To strengthen them, sit with your legs apart, then practice tightening and relaxing the muscles. If you are unsure of where the muscles are, try to contract them to stop the flow of urine. Once you master the technique, squeeze the muscles, hold, then release for three seconds at a time. Work up to a set of 30. As the muscles become stronger, your scrotum will rise and fall as you tighten and relax them.

See the light. If you want to delay your orgasm, focus on an imaginary light or candle, suggests Domeena Renshaw, M.D., director of the Sexual Dysfunction Clinic at Loyola University of Chicago Stritch School of Medicine. The light focus will momentarily divert your attention away from sex and extend your time to orgasm.

Get back to basics. "Couples stop doing the very things that brought them together in the first place," Dr. Seiler says. "They don't write each other little notes or send flowers. They don't give each other back rubs or go out on dates. You really have to work to keep the fun and play in the relationship. Without it, there won't be any fun and play in the bedroom."

Get a good sexual cookbook. If your sex life, like stale soda, has lost most of its fizz, try browsing through sex manuals or watching erotic videos together for new ideas, says Dr. Renshaw.

Keep your eyes open. "Sustained eye contact during sex breeds intimacy. Often, it's more intimate than kissing or holding hands," says Harrison Voigt, Ph.D., a clinical psychologist, sex therapist, and professor at the California Institute of Integral Studies in San Francisco. "It's a way to get people in touch with a powerful form of union that isn't physical."

Don't keep score. If you had sex four times last week and had an orgasm each time but had sex only once this week and did not have an orgasm, don't push to keep pace. "Frequency isn't as important as truly enjoying the sex that you do have," Dr. Zussman says.

The bedroom isn't a workplace. Your bedroom should be a place where you and your partner can retreat for intimate interludes. If it's cluttered with a computer, the television, a typewriter, and filing cabinets, it's an office. "There's something about disorder that distracts from romance. The bedroom should have a certain tranquillity," Dr. Zussman says.

SKIN CARE

Maintaining Your Youthful Look

Safeguarding your skin doesn't have to take much time at all. And despite the hype that surrounds big-name products, it really doesn't have to be complicated or expensive.

A good skin-care regimen just has to cleanse, moisturize, and protect your skin from the effects of too much time in the sun. If you use daily sun protection, doctors say that after a while your skin will repair some of the damage itself, leaving you looking younger and fresher.

Whether your skin is normal, oily, dry, or sun-damaged—and whether you're male or female—the watchword for cleansing is *gentle*, dermatologists say. Gentle cleansers and gentle handling. Why? Every time you rub, scrub, or otherwise yank your skin, you may loosen tiny fibers beneath the surface that promote firmness and a youthful look.

"Everything you do to your face adds a little age damage," says Albert M. Kligman, M.D., professor of dermatology at the University of Pennsylvania School of Medicine in Philadelphia.

Skin-Care Basics

Here's how to keep your skin fresh and young.

Choose gentle products. Forget harsh cleansers and astringents, says Seth L. Matarasso, M.D., assistant professor of dermatology at the University of California, San Francisco, School of Medicine. Inexpensive mild soaps like Purpose, Basis, Neutrogena, and Dove are all you need. If your skin's particularly dry, a thorough morning rinse with a soap substitute such as Cetaphil or no soap at all is fine.

Nuts to the nut scrubs. Washing with those ground-up nut scrubs and abrasive sponges is like taking kitchen cleansers to your skin, says Carole Walderman, a cosmetologist, an aesthetician, and president of Von Lee International School of Aesthetics and Makeup in Baltimore. The tiny scratches they leave behind inflame your skin and gather bacteria, promoting outbreaks.

Keep water temperature moderate. Use warm, not hot, water to rinse off your cleanser, says Leila Cohoon, a cosmetologist, aesthetician, and owner of Leila's Skin Care in Independence, Missouri. And don't bother with a cold-water splash to "close your pores" afterward. Pores do not open and close as commonly thought.

The Beauty of Moisturizers

Moisturizers do not add moisture to the skin. They do help retain the water that's left on your face and body after washing, which plumps up fine wrinkles and smooths the surface, says Dr. Matarasso. If you towel until you're bone-dry, any moisturizer—no matter how expensive—will just sit on top and feel greasy. But if you leave a damp film after you rinse, the moisturizer will help water get into the pores and sink deeper into your skin. If your skin is oily, you may not need a moisturizer; it may aggravate acne.

Here's what else you need to know about moisturizing:

Ask about AHAs. Alpha hydroxy acids (AHAs) are derived from food sources such as red wine, sour milk, and fruit. They improve sun-damaged skin by peeling dead cells off the skin's surface, exposing new cells underneath. Also, AHAs can smooth and firm the skin, filling in wrinkles.

AHAs are available over the counter in certain creams, lotions, and gels, most often in the form of glycolic acid. For general use on the face and neck, apply an 8 percent preparation in the morning and again at night, says Lorrie J. Klein, M.D., a dermatologist in private practice in Laguna Niguel, California. On the sensitive skin around the eyes, you can use a fragrance-free 5 percent cream.

Choose nonclogging lotions. If you have a tendency to break out, choose a moisturizer labeled "noncomedogenic," says Thomas Griffin, M.D., a dermatologist with Graduate Hospital of Philadelphia and clinical assistant professor of dermatology at the University of Pennsylvania School of Medicine. These products won't clog pores.

Check the pH. If your skin is sensitive, use a product that is the same acid balance (pH) as normal skin, which is in the range of pH 4.5 to 5.5, says Cohoon. "Many labels say 'pH-balanced,' but that might mean pH-balanced alkaline, which is not good for your skin. You want it to be pH-balanced acid for skin care."

To be sure, buy pH papers (such as pHydrion) from your skin-care salon and dip them in the product, Cohoon says. "The paper will change color, and you compare it with an enclosed color chart, which will show you what pH the moisturizer is."

Go lightly on the eye area. Use just a lightweight eye cream on the eye area during the day, says Walderman. Heavy eye creams tend to make makeup appear thick and pasty.

Get sunscreen protection. Sunscreen is the single most important age-erasing step in skin care. Using a sunscreen right now will pay youthful dividends for decades to come. The easiest way for women to add sunscreen is to use a lotion or cream-based sunscreen as their moisturizer, says Dr. Matarasso.

Be sure it's real protection. Choose a sunscreen or moisturizer-sunscreen combination with a sun protection factor (SPF) of at least 15, says Dr. Kligman. And sunscreens that block both the UVA and UVB forms of light (often called full-spectrum sunscreens) will offer you the best protection against both surface burning and the deeper tissue damage that causes wrinkles and sags, he says. Many cosmetic moisturizers trumpet their sun protection capabilities, but most contain very low-SPF sunscreens.

Remove makeup at bedtime. For a very thorough job, use a cleanser with petrolatum for removing makeup, says Marina Valmy, a cosmetician at the Christine Valmy Skin Care School in New York City. But only at night—petrolatum is too heavy for daytime cleansing or moisturizing, she says. Your favorite gentle soap is an option, too; just clean and rinse thoroughly. Add an overnight moisturizer if your skin tends toward dryness, or perhaps tretinoin (Retin-A) if you're actively battling sun damage.

Try a deep-pore cleanser. Three times a week, use a deep-pore cleanser and a soft facial brush for deep-cleaning your skin, says Walderman. These cleansers are labeled "deep-pore cleansers."

Sleep with a wrinkle-fighter. If sun damage has etched your skin with fine lines, ask your doctor about a prescription for Retin-A cream, says Jonathan Weiss, M.D., assistant clinical professor of dermatology at Emory University School of Medicine in Atlanta. "Retin-A is a wonderful product for sun damage. It can improve the yellowed appearance of the skin and make it more pink. But its greatest improvement is on wrinkles and age spots." He points out that the Food and Drug

Administration has not yet approved Retin-A for the treatment of sun-damaged and wrinkled skin, though the cream does seem effective.

Shaving the Edge Off the Years

For most men, skin care stops at the face, and men have a real advantage over women when it comes to facial aging. That's because shaving removes the top layer of dead cells that can make skin look dull. Shaving can give you a cleaner, younger appearance—but not if you leave your face looking like a war zone. These pointers will help.

Choose your weapon. The difference between an electric razor and any other kind of blade is just preference. If you opt for an electric razor, shave your face *before* you shower or wash, says John F. Romano, M.D., a dermatologist at New York Hospital–Cornell Medical Center in New York City. The natural oils that accumulate on your skin overnight act as a protective barrier between your face and the shaver. And to be kind to your skin, prep with a powder-based preshave rather than one containing alcohol, which can dry the skin, he says. If the blade's your weapon, read on.

Hydrate like mad. "Stand over the basin and splash a *lot* of lukewarm water on your skin first," says Dr. Matarasso. It will soften the hairs and make them easier to cut. A quick wetting of the skin isn't enough, he says.

Foam the runway. If razor burn is a problem, apply a layer of light lotion before you slap on your shaving cream, suggests Valmy.

Let it stand. After you lather on shaving cream, find a way to kill two or three minutes, says Dr. Matarasso. The cream needs time to soften your whiskers.

Don't stretch. Don't stretch your skin taut while you shave, that is. It's just another of those little torments that can make your skin sag and lose its firm tone after a few years, says Dr. Romano.

Go with the grain. Shave in the direction your beard grows, says Dr. Matarasso. If you shave against the grain, you'll cut the whiskers so short they'll spring back below the surface of the skin. Then when they start to regrow, they can cause folliculitis—those sore red "razor bumps."

Plug the oops. If you slip and nick yourself, reach for the old standby styptic pencil. Its main ingredient—aluminum chloride—coagulates blood and stops bleeding, Dr. Matarasso says, and it won't harm your skin.

Bag the bracer. If you're terribly attached to your aftershave, at least dilute it with distilled water, says Walderman. Most skin bracers irritate and dehydrate the skin, she says. Instead, use witch hazel or your wife's skin toner for that refreshing cheek-smack.

STRETCHING

Get Loose, Feel Good

Every once in a while, you find the time to stretch. When you do, you love the way it makes you feel—loose, limber, and relaxed. But those days are few and far between.

Usually you spend your time in overdrive, running from one activity to the next, with barely the time to sit and catch your breath, let alone stretch. You manage to squeeze in some walking or an aerobics class about three times a week, but that's about all you can usually handle. And stretching isn't really all that important anyway, right?

Wrong.

A general warm-up followed by regular stretching raises the temperature within our muscles and enables us to move smoothly and with a full range of motion—like we did when we were younger. In addition to relieving stress and tension, it improves flexibility, enhances performance, and helps prevent injuries.

Oh, Those Aging Muscles

As we get older, our muscles and joints tend to become tighter, says John Skowron, physical therapist at Raleigh Community Sports Medicine and Physical Therapy in North Carolina. That's because as we age, connective muscle tissues shorten. That makes it harder to do the activities we're used to, whether on the playing field or around the house, because our muscles just aren't ready.

Here's what happens: Any time you do an activity, whether it's

170

reaching up to paint a wall, carrying something down stairs, or going for a run, your muscles move. Certain muscles contract, or shorten, with movement, while the opposing muscles relax, or lengthen. When the muscles and surrounding elastic tissue that need to lengthen are too tight, they can't move the way you want them to, and you lose what health experts call your full range of motion; that is, your movement becomes restricted.

That can cause all kinds of trouble. Sometimes it prohibits you from participating in activities at all. Other times you can participate, but your performance is compromised. Then there are the times when this restricted movement leads to injury. When your body realizes it can't use a certain muscle group fully, it often tries to compensate by asking another muscle group to work harder than usual, a demand that can sometimes cause that part of the body to break down. And sometimes the muscles themselves are damaged—their tissues can tear, which is what happens when you "pull" a muscle.

Part of the reason we get tighter after age 30 has to do with our lifestyles, says Michael Kaplan, M.D., Ph.D., director of the Rehabilitation Team, a sports medicine and physical therapy clinic in Catonsville, Maryland. "Before they're 30, people tend not to have as many responsibilities. They often don't have the job that they have to do plus the house that they have to support, the kids they have to do things for," he says. Eventually, the sum of these responsibilities takes up most of their time. As a result, folks become less active and, unfortunately, less mobile and less flexible.

"There's no reason why people in their thirties and forties and even older can't have just as much flexibility as when they were younger—or even more flexibility," says Dr. Kaplan. "A 60-year-old can have more flexibility than a 20-year-old," if he works at it and stretches, he maintains.

Here's how it works. When you stretch a muscle, say, the hamstring muscle at the back of your leg, you place tension on it, and the muscle begins to lengthen. Initially, a stretch reflex inside the muscle tries to protect it from lengthening and asks the muscle to contract. But if the stretch is held long enough, then a structure located where tendons adjoin to muscles, called the Golgi tendon organ, sends a message that triggers the muscle to relax farther and lengthening continues.

That's what happens when you do the type of slow and steady stretching—called static stretching—that has generally been accepted as the right way to stretch these days. The idea is to move into the stretch slowly and gradually, hold it for 20 to 30 seconds, relax, and repeat. Research conducted at the Institute for Sports Medicine at Lenox Hill Hospital in New York City showed that the majority of muscle relaxation occurs within 20 seconds of stretching.

How to Do It Right

You can reap the benefits of stretching if you pay attention to your stretching technique. Here's what to keep in mind, according to the experts.

Warm up first. "You should warm up the muscle before you stretch it," says Lucille Smith, Ph.D., assistant professor at the Human Performance Laboratory at East Carolina University in Greenville, North Carolina. The general guideline is to warm up until you break a sweat. For activities involving the entire body, warm up with a brisk walk or light jog.

If you're going to be exercising only one area of your body, concentrate on that area. Warming up raises the temperature of the muscle and makes it less susceptible to injury. "When the muscle is heated up, it's more pliable," says Mark Taranta, a physical therapist and director of the Physical Therapy Practice in Philadelphia.

Go slow and steady. When you stretch, make it a slow and steady one, says William L. Cornelius, Ph.D., associate professor of physical education in the department of kinesiology, health promotion, and recreation at the University of North Texas in Denton. Don't bounce. Move into each stretch gradually until you feel tension in the muscle and connective tissue, he says. Hold that position for 20 to 30 seconds, relax, and do it again.

Be sure to breathe. "You really have to concentrate on your breathing," says Taranta. If you hold your breath, that can contribute to tensing of your muscles, whereas breathing helps relax them, he says.

Know that every little bit helps. You don't need to have 20 to 30 minutes to devote to stretching, says Dr. Kaplan. If you stretch your neck, shoulders, back, hips, and legs for 2 minutes each at 30-second intervals, that makes for a 10-minute stretching workout.

Get into a routine. It's important to be consistent about stretching, says Taranta. If you don't stretch regularly, it won't have much effect. Aim to stretch three times a week to start. Once you're in the habit, aim for every day, he says.

Pay attention to the temperature. When it's cold out, you may need to spend a little extra time stretching to get your muscles warm; when it's hot, you'll require a little less, says Taranta.

Do more in the morning. If you exercise in the morning or have to do physical labor first thing, take the time to warm up and stretch a little longer than usual. "Core temperature and body temperature probably would be lower and you'd probably be stiffer first thing in the morning versus later in the day, when you've already been moving around," says Dr. Smith.

Get in a group. Join or form a group of people interested in stretching together, says Dr. Kaplan. Yoga classes are one option. Or if you are part of a softball or volleyball team, make stretching together part of your practices and games, he says. "By yourself, you may lose incentive."

VITAMINS AND MINERALS

Life's Bare Necessities

Vitamins and minerals, the building blocks of youth and vitality, keep you alive and kicking. While nutritionists are only just beginning to understand everything they can do, it's known that vitamins and minerals give you what you need to perform physically, mentally, and emotionally. They rejuvenate and energize your cells. They make every single bodily process possible.

"As we age, our requirements for certain vitamins and minerals actually increase," says Jeffrey Blumberg, Ph.D., professor of nutrition and associate director of the Jean Mayer USDA Human Nutrition Research Center on Aging at Tufts University in Boston. "We tend to eat less food overall on a daily basis. So if your diet is already lacking a little in certain nutrients, as you get older, you stand a greater chance of widening that deficiency."

Low vitamin and mineral levels can lead to increased susceptibility to infection, slow healing, decreased mental capacity, and chronic fatigue, nutritionists say. The bottom line is obvious: To look, feel, and perform at your best, you can't make a habit of skimping on your vitamins and minerals.

Nutritionists divide the 13 essential vitamins into two groups based on their behavior in the body. Water-soluble vitamins—vitamin

C and the eight B vitamins (thiamin, riboflavin, niacin, B_6, pantothenic acid, B_{12}, biotin, and folate)—are short-lived, fast-acting compounds. The body quickly puts these vitamins to work assisting cells in chemical reactions and energy processing and usually excretes any excess.

Fat-soluble vitamins—A, D, E, and K—are found in the fatty parts of cells and regulate a wide variety of metabolic processes. They tend to be put in long-term storage and are then drawn upon as the body needs them.

Several vitamins have been singled out for their ability to slow down or even prevent the onset of age-related diseases, like heart disease and cancer, and potentially slow the aging process itself. These vitamins—C, E, and beta-carotene (a substance the body converts to vitamin A)—are known as antioxidants for their ability to neutralize destructive oxygen-derived particles believed to initiate many disease processes.

Like vitamins, minerals help keep the body functioning. But unlike vitamins, they are inorganic and not metabolized by the body. Instead, they act more like building blocks, providing structure to bones and teeth, serving as major components in blood, skin, and tissue, and keeping our bodily fluids in balance. Some minerals are stored in the body, on reserve to replace those we lose in our urine and sweat. If we don't replenish our mineral stores as rapidly as they are being depleted, we run the risk of developing diseases such as iron-deficiency anemia and osteoporosis.

Getting the right amount of these essential nutrients takes planning, and to make that task easier, the National Research Council's Food and Nutrition Board has established guidelines for vitamin and mineral consumption. They're called Recommended Dietary Allowances (RDAs).

RDAs are the amount of a nutrient judged to be adequate for the average healthy person. What about people who want to achieve superior health? "A growing body of evidence indicates a direct link between increased longevity and improved overall health when certain vitamin and mineral intakes exceed the RDAs," says Dr. Blumberg. "This suggests that perhaps the RDAs are inadequate for the changing needs of the aging adult."

Research is in the works to determine the exact levels of each vitamin and mineral needed for optimal health. Until such results are found, doctors say that your goal at the very least should be to shoot for 100 percent of the RDAs for every essential vitamin and mineral, especially if you lead an active life.

Food: Our Best Source

Here are some tips for getting the maximum vitamin and mineral content from the foods you eat—and for the least amount of calories.

Go for the basics. "Concentrate on eating from the five basic food groups—fruits, vegetables, lean meats and legumes, grains and cereals, and low-fat or nonfat dairy products," says Diane Grabowski-Nepa, R.D., a nutrition educator at the Pritikin Longevity Center in Santa Monica, California. "Junk food just gives your body empty calories that are devoid of vitamins and minerals."

Focus on fruits and veggies. "You should eat a minimum of five good-size servings of fruits and vegetables every day," says Grabowski-Nepa. "In most cases, the darkest or most vibrantly colored fruits and vegetables have the richest vitamin and mineral content." Color your diet with such perennial favorites as cantaloupe, oranges, peaches, tomatoes, spinach, yams, and carrots.

Eat 'em raw. Cooking food draws out or destroys many vitamins and minerals, so whenever you can, try to eat fruits, vegetables, and grains in their natural raw or unprocessed state or minimally cooked. Be aware that boiling tends to leach out more nutrients than other cooking methods, says Grabowski-Nepa; she recommends steaming or microwaving instead.

Trap nutrients. Exposure to air can rob vitamins and minerals from food. So can sunlight when it penetrates glass bottles or cellophane wrap. Grabowski-Nepa recommends using airtight, opaque containers. For long-term storage of foods or juices, try freezing. It keeps nutrients intact for a long time.

Watch out for medications. Certain drugs and over-the-counter medications can interfere with the body's vitamin and mineral stores. Aspirin, laxatives, diuretics, antibiotics, antidepressants, and antacids can accelerate the excretion of some vitamins and minerals or impede their absorption. If you are taking any of these medications, consult your doctor before quitting or trying alternatives.

The Scoop on Supplements

Here are some guidelines for selecting and using supplements.

Go multi. A safe and beneficial supplement would be a once-a-day-type multivitamin with minerals, says Grabowski-Nepa. Such a supplement should contain a mixture of all or most of the essential vitamins and minerals and contain approximately 100 percent of the RDAs for each.

Take care with single supplements. In most cases, you probably don't need extra doses of specific vitamins and minerals if you are taking a multivitamin and eating right. Exceptions would be if you are under a doctor's treatment for a deficiency or if you are seeking antioxidant protection by taking extra vitamin C, vitamin E, and beta-carotene. Otherwise, avoid single supplements—especially vitamin A, vitamin D, and iron, says Paul R. Thomas, R.D., Ed.D., a staff scientist with the Food and Nutrition Board of the National Academy of Sciences in Washington, D.C. These nutrients are toxic in high doses.

Don't forget your calcium. Calcium is vital for bone strength and for staving off osteoporosis—the bone-thinning disease that creeps up on many women after menopause. But studies show that most women don't get the recommended 1,000 milligrams a day before menopause and 1,000 to 1,500 milligrams thereafter. That's why calcium supplements are recommended for women as added protection against bone loss.

The most easily absorbed calcium supplements are those made with calcium citrate, says Margo Denke, M.D., assistant professor of medicine at the Center for Human Nutrition at the University of Texas Southwestern Medical Center at Dallas and a member of the nutrition committee of the American Heart Association. They are more easily absorbed by the body than supplements made with calcium carbonate, she says.

If you prefer to get your calcium from inexpensive over-the-counter antacid tablets made from calcium carbonate, it's best to take them with meals, says Clifford Rosen, M.D., director of the Maine Center for Osteoporosis Research and Education in Bangor. The acid your body produces when you eat will break down the calcium carbonate and allow it to be absorbed, he says. Aluminum-containing antacids like Gelusil, Maalox, and Mylanta are not recommended as regular supplements. Your best choices are Tums and Rolaids—both aluminum-free.

Look into generics. Generic and store brands are typically comparable in quality to big-name brands, says Dr. Thomas. In fact, generics are often produced by the same manufacturers as the big-name brands but cost a lot less.

Forget "super-supplements." You may see "high potency" or "extra strength" on labels. These products typically contain levels of vitamins and minerals that greatly exceed the RDAs and may be hazardous, says Dr. Thomas. Or you may just end up excreting the excess, in which case you're wasting your money.

Say no to gimmicks. Phrases like "anti-stress formula" are bogus, says Dr. Thomas, and although "time-released" and "effervescent" are legitimate descriptors, in some supplements these qualities may not matter. For example, effervescence in calcium may be helpful, but it is not needed in vitamin C. Check with your physician or nutrition professional.

Avoid multiple dosages. If the label tells you to take more than one a day, check the total amount to see how it compares with the RDA. If it's way over, this may be a ploy to get you to shell out more money, Dr. Thomas says.

Pop 'em with a meal. As a general rule, supplements will be absorbed more efficiently by the body if they are taken during a meal rather than on an empty stomach, says Dr. Thomas. They will also break down better if they're taken with water or some other beverage.

Check the expiration date. When shopping for supplements, make sure an expiration date is on the label. If the date has passed or is just around the corner, find a bottle with a longer shelf life.

Keep 'em in a cool, dry place. Light, heat, and moisture can rob supplements of their potency. Because of this, a kitchen cabinet, away from the heat of the stove, is probably a better place to keep your supplements than on the windowsill or in a bathroom medicine chest. The refrigerator is another good storage place. Try to use a nontransparent container and always secure the cap tightly.

INDEX

A

A-B-C technique, optimism and, 149–50
Achromycin (Rx), 4
Acid balance (pH), 168
Adventure, seeking, 87–89
Adversity, coping with, 149
Aerobic exercise, 91–92
  as age rejuvenator, 90–93
  classes, 90
  cholesterol levels and, 91
  guidelines for, 92–93
  in managing
    cellulite, 19
    double chin, 22
    impotence, 47
    menopause, 90
    premenstural syndrome, 90
    Type A personality, 72
    wrinkles, 84
  types of, 90–91
  weight loss and, 60
Affirmations, as age rejuvenator, 94–96
Aftershave, 169
Age rejuvenators
  adventure, 87–89
  aerobic exercise, 90–93
  affirmations, 94–96

altruism, 97–100
antioxidants, 101–4
breast care, 105–8
confidence and self-esteem, 109–11
fiber, 112–15
friendship, 119–21
goals, 122–24
hormone replacement therapy, 125–28
humor, 129–32
learning, 133–35
low-fat diet, 136–39
massage, 140–42
medical checkup, 143–47
optimism, 148–50
relaxation, 151–54
religion and spirituality, 155–58
resistance training, 159–62
sex, 163–65
skin care, 166–69
stretching, 170–73
vitamins and minerals, 174–78
volunteering, 97–100
water intake, 116–18
Age-related problems
  age spots, 3–5
  arthritis, 6–9

Age-related problems *(continued)*
    back pain, 10–13
    burnout, 14–17
    cellulite, 18–20
    double chin, 21–23
    fatigue, 24–26
    foot problems, 27–30
    gray hair, 31–33
    hair loss, 34–37
    hearing loss, 38–41
    high blood pressure, 42–45
    impotence, 46–48
    menopause, 49–52
    osteoporosis, 53–56
    overweight, 57–60
    prostate problems, 61–63
    stress, 64–67
    television addiction, 68–70
    Type A personality, 71–73
    varicose veins, 74–76
    vision changes, 77–80
    wrinkles, 81–84
Age spots, 3–5
AHAs, 19, 81–82, 167
Alcohol
    diuretic effect of, 117
    estrogen and, 107
    fatigue and, 26
    high blood pressure and, 45
    impotence and, 47–48
    osteoporosis and, 54–55
    prostate problems and, 63
Alpha hydroxy acids (AHAs), 19,
        81–82, 167
Altruism
    as age rejuvenator, 97–100
    burnout and, 16–17, 99–100
Aluminum chloride, for skin care, 169
American Massage Therapy
        Association (AMTA), 141–42
Anger
    impotence and, 48
    Type A personality and, 72–73
Antacids, 177
Antibiotics, 4
Anticonvulsants, 55

Antidepressants, 47
Anti-inflammatory steroids, 55
Antioxidants, 80, 101–4, 175
Antipsychotic drugs, 4, 47
Arteries, hardening of, 101
Arthritis, 6–9
Astroglide, 51–52
Atherosclerosis, 101
Athlete's foot, 30

B

Back pain, 10–13
Baking soda, athlete's foot and, 30
Balding, 34–37
Barbita (Rx), 55
Bath, hot, 63, 66
Beef, 138
Ben-Gay, 9
Benign prostatic hyperplasia (BPH), 62
Bergamot oil, age spots and, 4
Beta-carotene, 80, 103–4, 175
Beta hydroxy acid, 82
Biopsy, endometrial, 128
Birth control pills, 43
Blisters, 29
Blood flow
    dietary fat and, 47
    exercise and, 40
    smoking and, 12, 40, 151–52
Blood pressure, high, 42–45, 152
Blood pressure monitors, 43
Blood sugar, 101
Blue Cross and Blue Shield study on
        spine operations, 13
Body fat, 160. *See also* Overweight
Bone
    problems, 13, 53–56, 144
    strength, maintaining, 160
BPH, 62
Bread, whole-grain, 114, 137
Breast
    cancer, 105, 107, 126
    care, 105–8
    sag, 107–8
    self-exam, 105–6, 127–28

Breathing
  calming effect of, 153
  in exercising, 172
  in resistance training, 161
  in stress management, 66
Bunions, 29
Burnout
  as age-related problem, 14–17
  perfectionism and, 15–16
  volunteering and, 16–17, 99–100

C

Caffeine, 26, 40, 117
Calcitonin (Rx), 55
Calcium
  menopause and, 50–51
  osteoporosis and, 13, 53–55
  sources of, 12
  supplements, 177
Calluses, 28–29
Calories, 103, 160
Cancer
  breast, 105, 107, 126
  hair coloring and, 33
  low-fat diet and, 106–7
  melanoma, 5
  preventing, 106–7
  prostate, 62, 144–45
  testicular, 145
Carbohydrates, 58–59, 66, 152
CAT, 54
Cataracts, 78–80
Cellex-C, 82
Cellulite, 18–20
Cereals, 113, 137
Cheese, low-fat, 137–38
Chicken, 137–38
Chin, double, 21–23
Chiropractic treatment, 13
Chlorpromazine (Rx), 4
Cholesterol levels
  aerobic exercise and, 91
  fiber and, 113
  free radicals and, 101–2

high-density lipoprotein and, 91
low-density lipoprotein and, 91,
  101–2, 113
prostate problems and, 62–63
testosterone and, 62–63
Cibacalcin (Rx), 55
Cigarettes. *See* Smoking
Circulation problems, 30
Coffee, 26, 40, 117
Collagen, 83–84
Computerized axial tomography
  (CAT), 54
Conditioner, hair, 32, 37
Confidence, building, 109–11
Cooking food, 138, 176
Coping skills, 149
Corns, 28–29
Cortisol, 140
Cortisone (Rx), 55
Cortone Acetate (Rx), 55
Cosmetics, double chin and, 22
Cosmetic surgery, 20, 23
Cravings, food, 59–60

D

Dehydration, 26
Depressants, 55
Depression, 150
DEXA, 54
DHT, 35
Diabetes, 30, 152
Diabetic retinopathy, 79
Diet. *See also* Low-fat diet; *specific foods*
  cooking food and, 138, 176
  cravings and, 59–60
  dieting and, 57
  effects of, on
    arthritis, 8
    cellulite, 19
    fatigue, 25–26
    hearing loss, 40
    impotence, 47
    menopause, 50
    overweight, 58–60
    vision changes, 80

Diet *(continued)*
energizing, 25–26
fiber in, 45, 75, 114–15
food groups and, 176
grazing and, 59
junk-food, 25
magnesium in, 45
potassium in, 44–45
salty food in, 117
skipping meals and, 26
snacking and, 26
sodium in, 44
splurges and, 59
sugar in, 26, 59
water-rich food in, 117
Dietary fat. *See also* Low-fat diet
blood flow and, 47
calories and, 160
flavor and, 137–39
in food, 136–37
in fruits, 136–37
in vegetables, 136–37
weight loss and, 58
Dieting, 57
Digestion, 103
Dihydrotestosterone (DHT), 35
Dilantin (Rx), 55
Diuretics, 4, 47, 55
Drinking. *See* Alcohol; Water intake
Dr. Scholl's ingrown toenail reliever, 30
Drugs. *See* Over-the-counter products; Prescription drugs; *specific types*
Dual energy x-ray absorptiometry (DEXA), 54

E

Earplugs, for hearing loss prevention, 39
Ear problems, 38–41
EarthCorps, 99
Earthwatch, 99
Education, continued, 133–35
Eldoquin, 5

Electrolytes, 118
Emotional needs, 58
Estrogen, 51–52, 106–7, 126
Exercise. *See also* Aerobic exercise; Stretching
avoiding excessive, 103–4
blood flow and, 40
breathing during, 172
in confidence-building, 109–10
facial, 84
group, 93, 173
Kegel, 164
in managing
arthritis, 8–9
fatigue, 25
high blood pressure, 44
menopause, 50
osteoporosis, 55–56
overweight, 60
prostate problems, 63
stress, 65–66
varicose veins, 75
with partner, 93
protective equipment and, 9
for relaxation, 153–54
resistance training, 159–62
rest and, 9, 11
rolling, 28
running, 75
walking, 11, 25, 67
warmup before, 92–93, 172
water intake and, 117–18
weight-bearing, 91, 160
weight lifting, 9, 19, 56, 75
weight loss and, 60
Eye
creams, 168
problems, 77–80

F

Family medical history, 127, 144
Fat. *See* Body fat; Dietary fat
Fatigue, 24–26
alternative approaches to managing, 26

Fat-soluble vitamins, 175
Feedback, positive, 16
Fiber, 112–13
    as age rejuvenator, 112–15
    cholesterol levels and, 113
    in diet, 45, 75, 114–15
    in fruits, 114–15
    high blood pressure and, 45
    pills, 115
    varicose veins and, 75
    in vegetables, 114
Fish, 137
Flexibility of muscles, 171
Fluids. *See* Water intake
Food. *See* Diet; *specific types*
    cooking, 138, 176
    groups, 176
Foot problems, 27–30
Fracture, penile, 48
Freckles, age spots vs., 3
Free radicals, 82, 101–4
Freezing treatment for age spots, 5
Friendships, 119–21
Fruits
    dietary fat in, 136–37
    fiber in, 114–15
    minerals in, 176
    vitamins in, 176
Fungus, foot, 30
Furosemide (Rx), 55

G

Gelusil, 177
Genetics, diseases and, 74, 144–45
Glaucoma, 78
Glucose, 101
Glycolic acid, 81
Goals, setting
    as age rejuvenator, 122–24
    hierarchy in, 110
    realistic, 72
Golgi tendon organ, 171
Gradient stockings, varicose veins
        and, 76
Grazing, 59

H

Habitat for Humanity International,
        99
Hair
    coloring, 5, 32–33, 37
    conditioner, 32, 37
    cutting, 22, 32, 37
    gray, 31–33
    highlighting, 32
    lifts, 36
    loss, 34–37
    transplants, 36
Hair-lifts, 36
Hand exerciser, 66
Harvard study on
    fitness, 91
    smoking, 80
    Type A personality, 72
HDL, 91
Hearing loss, 38–41
Heart disease, 145, 152
Heart rate, raising, 72
Heat treatment for
    arthritis, 9
    foot pain, 28
Heel pain, 27–28
Herbs, 137
Heredity, diseases and, 74, 144–45
High blood pressure, 42–45, 152
High-density lipoprotein (HDL),
        91
HIV, 141
Hormonal changes, 49–52. *See also*
        specific hormones
Hormone replacement therapy
        (HRT)
    as age rejuvenator, 125–28
    breast sag and, 108
    decisions about, 125–27
    guidelines, 127–28
    menopause and, 51–52
    osteoporosis and, 56
Hot flashes, 52, 126
HRT. *See* Hormone replacement
        therapy

Humor
  as age rejuvenator, 129–32
  pain and, 129–30
  as relaxation technique, 152
  in stress management, 66, 89
Hydrocortisone (Rx), 55
Hydroquinone, 5
Hypertension, 42–45, 152

I

Ice treatment for
  arthritis, 9
  back pain, 12–13
  foot pain, 28
Imagery, 153
Impotence, 46–48
Ingrown toenails, 30
Insulin, 59
Intimacy, 165
Inventory, taking personal, 110

J

Joint problems, 6–9
Journal
  food, 144
  spiritual, 158
  in stress management, 152
Junk food, 25

K

Kegel exercises, 164
Key-Pred 50 (Rx), 55
K-Y Jelly, 51–52

L

Labels, food, 44, 47, 114
Lactic acid, 81
Laser treatment, 5, 83
Lasix (Rx), 55
Laughter. *See* Humor
Laxatives, 117
LDL, 91, 101–2, 113
Learning, as age rejuvenator, 133–35

Leg problems, 74–76
Legumes, 137
Lifting technique, correct, 11
Liver spots, 3–5
Locoid (Rx), 55
Log, food, 144
Low-density lipoprotein (LDL), 91,
  101–2, 113
Low-fat diet
  as age rejuvenator, 136–39
  arthritis and, 8
  cancer and, 106–7
  flavoring and, 137–39
  foods in, 136–37
  prostate problems and, 63
  weight loss and, 58–59
Lubricants, vaginal, 51–52
Lumbar roll, 12
Lysol, athlete's foot and, 30

M

Maalox, 177
Macular degeneration, 79
Magnesium, 45
Makeup, double chin and, 22
Mammogram, 128
Massage, 140–41
  as age rejuvenator, 140–42
  in cellulite management, 19
  in fatigue management, 26
  guidelines, 141–42
Mattress, back pain and, 12
Meals, skipping, 26
Meats, 137–38
Medical checkup, 92, 143–47, 161
Medications. *See* Over-the-counter
    products; Prescription drugs;
    specific types
Meditation, 26, 66, 153, 157
Melanex, 5
Melanoma, 5
Menopause, 49–52, 90, 146
Menstrual records, 127
Milk fat, 138
Minerals, 174–78. *See also specific types*
Minoxidil, 35

Moisturizer, skin, in
  cellulite management, 19
  corn and callus management, 29
  skin care, 167–69
  wrinkle management, 82
Moleskin, 29
Monosaturated fat, 136
Multivitamin, 26, 176
Muscles
  calories and, 160
  flexibility of, 171
  stretching and, 154, 170–72
Music, in stress management, 66–67
Musk, age spots and, 4
Mylanta, 177

N

Negative thinking, 149–50
Nice 'n Easy hair coloring, 5
Nicotine. *See* Smoking
Nip-and-tuck surgery, 20
Nitrogen, liquid, age spots and, 5
Noise levels, managing, 39–40
Nutrients, 176. *See also specific types*
Nutritional information, 114

O

Oat bran, 113–14
Obesity. *See* Overweight
Oil, cooking, 138
Oil of Olay's Age-Defying Series, 82
Omega-3 fatty acids, 8
Optimism, as age rejuvenator, 148–50
Orgasm, 165
Osteoarthritis, 7–9
Osteoporosis
  as age-related problem, 53–56
  alcohol and, 54–55
  calcium and, 13, 53–55
  exercise in managing, 55–56
  genetics and, 144
  hormone replacement therapy and,
    56
  smoking and, 54, 56
Outgro solution, 30

Over-the-counter products. *See also*
    specific types
  fiber pills, 115
  hair loss, 35
  ingrown toenail, 30
  mineral and vitamin body stores
    and, 176
Overweight
  as age-related problem, 57–60
  arthritis and, 8
  diet and, 58–60
  dieting and, 57
  double chin and, 22
  exercise and, 60
  high blood pressure and, 42–44,
    152
  impotence and, 47
  varicose veins and, 75
  weight loss and, 58–60

P

Pain
  arthritis, 6–9
  back, 10–13
  foot, 27–28
  heel, 27–28
  humor and, 129–30
  varicose veins, 74–76
Pasta, 114, 137
Penile fracture, 48
Perfectionism, burnout and, 15–16
Peroxide, 5
Personality problems, 71–73
Pets, companionship of, 121
pH, 168
Phenobarbital (Rx), 55
Phenytoin (Rx), 55
pHydrion, 168
Physical activity. *See* Exercise
Physical examination, 92, 143–47, 161
Phytoestrogens, 106–7
Pill, birth control, 43
PMS, 90
Polyunsaturated fat, 136–37
Pork, 138
Positive talk, 94–96

Positive thinking, 95, 148–50
Posture, back pain and, 12
Potassium, 44–45
Potatoes, 115, 137
Poultry, 137–38
Prayer, making time for, 157
Prednisone (Rx), 55
Premenstrual syndrome (PMS), 90
Prescription drugs. *See also specific types*
    as causes of
        age spots, 4
        fatigue, 26
        impotence, 47
        osteoporosis, 55
    in treating
        age spots, 5
        hair loss, 35
        high blood pressure, 43, 47
        thyroid problems, 55
Prioritizing, in stress management, 65
Progressive relaxation, 154
Propecia (Rx), 35
Prostate
    cancer, 62, 144–45
    problems, 61–63
    prostatitis, 62
Protein, 58, 152
Psoralens, 3–4
Pubococcygeus muscles, 164

R

Recommended Dietary Allowances
    (RDAs), 102, 175
Relationships with friends, 119–21
Relaxation, 17, 151–54
Religion, 96, 155–58
Renova (Rx), 83
Replens, 51–52
Resistance training, 159–62. *See also Weight lifting*
Rest
    back pain and, 13
    exercise and, 9, 11
Retin-A (Rx), 5, 83–84, 108, 168–69

Retin-A Micro (Rx), 83
Rheumatoid arthritis, 7–8
Rice, brown, 115, 137
Rogaine, 35
Rolling exercise, 28
Roughage. *See* Fiber
Running, 75

S

Salicylic acid, foot problems and, 29
Salt, 44
Salty food, 117
Saturated fat, 136
Scalp reduction, 36
Sclerotherapy, 76
Seasonings, food, 137
Self-acceptance, 157
Self-esteem, 109–11
Self-exam, breast, 105–6, 127–28
Self-improvement, as age
    rejuvenator, 133–35
Sex, 163–65
    problems, 46–48
Sexual relationships, 48
Shaving, skin care and, 169
Shellfish, 137
Shoes
    athlete's foot and, 30
    back pain and, 12
Skin
    care, 166–69
    cream. *See* Moisturizer, skin
    problems
        age spots, 3–5
        cellulite, 18–20
        wrinkles, 81–84
Sleep, 152
Smoking
    antioxidants and, 103
    blood flow and, 12, 40, 151–52
    Harvard study on, 80
    high blood pressure and, 45
    impotence and, 46
    menopause and, 50
    osteoporosis and, 54, 56

varicose veins and, 75
vision changes and, 80
Snacking, 26
Sodium, 44
Solar lentigos, 3–5
SPF, 4, 20, 84, 168
Spices, 137
Spicy foods, effects of, 52, 63
Spirituality, 96, 155–58
Splints, 29
Sports, competitive, 111
Sports drinks, 118
Steroids, 55. *See also specific types*
Stress
  as age-related problem, 64–67
  effects of, 64, 72
  high blood pressure and, 43
  hormones produced by, 72
  managing, with
    breathing, 66
    carbohydrates, 66
    exercise, 65–66
    hot bath, 66
    humor, 66, 89
    journal writing, 152
    meditation, 66
    music, 66–67
    planning tasks, 65–66
    prioritizing, 65
    saying "no," 65, 67
Stretching, 170
  as age rejunvenator, 170–73
  back pain and, 11
  before exercise, 92–93
  early morning, 11
  foot or heel pain and, 28
  guidelines, 172–73
  muscles and, 154, 170–72
  for relaxation, 154
Stretch marks, 108
Stripping, surgical, varicose veins
  and, 76
Styptic pencil, 169
Sugar, 26, 59, 139
Sunglasses, in vision change
  prevention, 80

Sun protection factor (SPF), 4, 20, 84,
  168
Sunscreen, 4, 20, 84, 168
Supplements, vitamin and mineral,
  26, 176–78
Support groups, 51
Support hose, varicose veins and, 76
Surgical treatment
  for cellulite, 20
  for double chin, 23
  for hair loss, 36
  for varicose veins, 76
Sweet potatoes, 137

T

Tanning cream, in cellulite
  management, 19
Television addiction, as age-related
  problem, 68–70
Testicular cancer, 145
Testosterone, 47–48, 62–63
Tetracycline (Rx), 4
Thorazine (Rx), 4
Thrill-seeking, 87–89
Thyroid medications, 55
Toenails, ingrown, 30
Touch Research Institute study on
  massage, 141
Transplants, hair, 36
Tretinoin (Rx), 5, 83–84, 108,
  168–69
Trichloroacetic acid, 5
Turkey, 138
Type A personality, 71–73
Type B personality, 72
Tyrosine, 82

U

Ultraviolet radiation (UVA and UVB),
  80, 84
Ultress hair coloring, 5
Urination, frequent, 63
UVA, 80, 84
UVB, 80, 84

V

Vacations, in burnout prevention, 17
Vaginal dryness, 51, 126
Varicose veins, 74–76
Vegetables
   breast cancer and, 107
   dietary fat in, 136–37
   fiber in, 114
   minerals in, 176
   prostate problems and, 63
   vitamins in, 176
Vision changes, 77–80
Visualization, 124, 153
Vitamin C, 80, 82, 104, 175
Vitamin D, 54–55
Vitamin E, 80, 103–4, 175
Vitamins, 174–78. *See also specific types*
Volunteering
   as age rejuvenator, 97–100
   burnout and, 16–17, 99–100

W

Walking, 11, 25, 67
Warmup before exercise, 92–93, 172

Water intake
   as age rejuvenator, 116–18
   dehydration and, 26
   exercise and, 117–18
   fatigue and, 26
   maintaining, 116–18
   prostate problems and, 63
   varicose veins and, 75
   weight loss and, 59
Water pills, 4
Water-rich food, 117
Water-soluble vitamins, 174–75
Weight-bearing exercise, 91, 160
Weight lifting, 9, 19, 56, 75. *See also* Resistance training
Weight loss, 58–60
Wheat bran, 113–14
Wishful thinking, 95
Wrinkles, 81–84, 126

Y

Yoga, 26

Z

Zinc, 63, 82